Chair
Yoga

of related interest

Curves, Twists and Bends
A Practical Guide to Pilates for Scoliosis
Annette Wellings and Alan Herdman
ISBN 9781848190252

The Healing Power of Mudras
The Yoga of the Hands
Rajendar Menen
ISBN 9781848190436

Yoga Therapy for Every Special Child
Meeting Needs in a Natural Setting
Nancy Williams
Illustrated by Leslie White
ISBN 9781848190276

A Tai Chi Imagery Workbook
Spirit, Intent, and Motion
Martin Mellish
ISBN 9781848190290

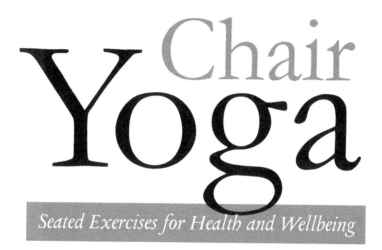

Chair Yoga

Seated Exercises for Health and Wellbeing

Edeltraud Rohnfeld

Translated by Anne Oppenheimer

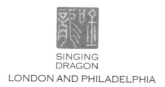

SINGING
DRAGON
LONDON AND PHILADELPHIA

This English translation of *Yoga auf dem Stuhl* (first published in German in 2004) is
published by arrangement with Verlag Via Nova, 36100 Petersberg, Germany

English language edition first published in 2012
by Singing Dragon
an imprint of Jessica Kingsley Publishers
116 Pentonville Road
London N1 9JB, UK
and
400 Market Street, Suite 400
Philadelphia, PA 19106, USA

www.singingdragon.com

Library of Congress Cataloging in Publication Data
Rohnfeld, Edeltraud.
[Yoga auf dem Stuhl. English.]
Chair yoga : seated exercises for health and wellbeing / Edeltraud Rohnfeld
; translated by Anne Oppenheimer.
p. cm.
Includes index.
ISBN 978-1-84819-078-8 (alk. paper)
1. Yoga. 2. Sitting position. I. Oppenheimer, Anne. II. Title.
B132.Y6R6513 2012
613.7'046--dc22
2011010421

British Library Cataloguing in Publication Data
A CIP catalogue record for this book is available from the British Library

ISBN 978 1 84819 078 8

Printed and bound in Great Britain

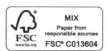

For Erika Hammerström and a very particular angel

ACKNOWLEDGEMENTS

Many people have contributed to the writing of this book. First and foremost I wish to thank Teresa Dunne, my friend of many years, without whose patience and support I would not have been able to write this book. In equal measure I thank my friend Eva Jabs and my neighbours Bettina Grandt and Heidi Kull for their great computer know-how.

I thank my yoga teachers Asha and Keshav Rekai for my fine training, and also the late Swami Dr Gitananda, who developed it. Further thanks go to Erika Hammerström, who set me on the path of 'Chair Yoga', and to all the senior citizens who have so far accompanied me along it.

Thanks also to Irma Dilba-Burnautzki for her great support and for setting a positive example of how to write a book.

Finally I wish to thank my editors Klaus Scheddel and Sonka Hecker, who had faith that my book would become a reality and helped to realize this dream.

Last of all I thank my parents, siblings and everyone else in my family. Very special thanks are due to my sister, Andrea Rohnfeld, who first showed me yoga exercises many years ago. I thank her and her friend Werner 'Spencer' Bläss for leading me onto the yoga path.

Yoga DVDs (in English and German) by the author can be ordered by phone on (00 353) 86 365 6209, from www.yoga-clare.com or by e-mail.

E-mail: edel.rohnfeld@freenet.de or edelireland@gmail.com

CONTENTS

Introduction   *13*
What is chair yoga?   13
Why do yoga today?   15
The exercises: General rules   18

1. The Importance of Breathing Practice   *19*
Pranayama – control of the breath   19

The breathing exercises: *Mahat Mudra* – breathing into the
    separate parts of the lungs   22
1.1 The inferior front part of the lungs (*Adham Pranayama*)   22
1.2 The middle front part of the lungs (*Madhyam Pranayama*)   23
1.3 The superior front part of the lungs (*Adhyam Pranayama*)   24
1.4 Full yogic breathing (*Mahat Yoga Pranayama*)   25

The breathing exercises: Breathing into the side and back
    parts of the lungs   26
1.5 The lower side and back region of the lungs   26
1.6 The middle part of the side and back region of the lungs   27
1.7 The upper side and back region of the lungs   28
1.8 *Savitri Pranayama*   29
1.9 Alternate nostril breathing (*Surya Bhedana Pranayama*)   31

2. Exercises for the Feet and Toes   *33*
2.1 Raising the heels   35
2.2 Rocking on the soles of the feet   36
2.3 Rolling the feet   37
2.4 Waking up the feet   38
2.5 Loosening and spreading the toes   39
2.6 Clenching the toes   40

2.7 Stretching the feet 41

    Variation 41

2.8 Walking on tiptoe and on the heels 42

3. Exercises for the Legs   43

3.1 Pushing the knees sideways 44

3.2 Massaging the legs 45

3.3 Bending the legs 46

3.4 Making circles with the heels 47

3.5 Wind-releasing exercise (*Pavanmuktasana*) 48

3.6 Clapping under the legs 49

3.7 Bicycling 50

    Variation for advanced students with good abdominal muscles 50

3.8 Stimulating lymph flow in the lower part of the body 51

    Variation for advanced students with good abdominal muscles 51

3.9 Boat pose 53

    Variation 1 (*Navasana*) 53

    Variation 2 (*Nava Kriya*) 53

4. Exercises for the Fingers, Hands and Wrists   55

4.1 Interlacing the fingers (an exercise to develop skill) 57

4.2 Pressing the fingertips together 58

4.3 Locking the fingers together 59

4.4 Pressing the palms of the hands together 60

4.5 Moving all the fingers separately 61

4.6 Making circles with the fingers 62

4.7 Fingertips touching 63

4.8 Spreading out the fingers/making fists 64

4.9 Opening the hands 65

4.10 The bud 66

4.11 Exercise for the wrists 67

4.12 Bending the wrists 68

4.13 Stretching the hands 69

    Variation 69

5. Exercises for the Arms   71

5.1 Making circles with the arms 73

    Variation 1 73

    Variation 2 74

5.2 Extending the elbows 75

5.3 Widening the chest 76

5.4 Relaxing the ribcage 77

5.5 Crossing your arms 78

5.6 Stretching the arms 79

5.7 Harmonizing exercise 80

5.8 'PAH' exercise – loosening up the arms 83

5.9 Mountain pose – upward stretch 84

    Variation 1 84

    Variation 2 85

5.10 Clapping your hands above your head 86

5.11 Stretching the arms and letting them go 87

5.12 Pushing the walls apart 88

5.13 Pushing weights 89

6. Exercises for the Back 91

6.1 Dance pose (*Natarajasana*) 93

6.2 Twisting forward bend 94

    Variation 1 94

    Variation 2 95

6.3 Half spinal twist (*Matsyendra Asana*) 96

    Variation 97

6.4 Tiger breathing 98

6.5 Back and arm extension 99

    Variation 1 99

    Variation 2 100

6.6 Spinal twist with arms bent 101

    Variation 101

6.7 Spinal twist with outstretched arms 103

6.8 Lateral extension 105

6.9 Back flexion with leg extension 106

7. Exercises for the Shoulders, Throat and Neck 107

7.1 Propeller 109

7.2 Dropping the shoulders 110

7.3 Circling with the shoulders 111

    Variation 1 111

    Variation 2 112

7.4 Massaging the shoulders 113

7.5 Shoulder stretches 114

7.6 Head leaning to one side 115

7.7 Turning the head slowly (*Brahma Mudra*) 116

    Variation 1 116

    Variation 2 117

7.8 Shoulder rotation 118

■ **8. Standing Exercises (Some With a chair, Some Without) 119**

8.1 Half (or crescent) moon — 121
8.2 The crane — 123
8.3 Walking with a spring in your step — 125
8.4 Circling the knees — 126
8.5 Circling the hips — 127
8.6 Circling the upper body — 128
8.7 Variation on standing twist (*Dola Dolati*, 'pendulum') — 129

■ **9. Exercises for Both Sides of the Brain — 131**

9.1 'Clang' exercise — 133
9.2 'Gong' exercise — 134
9.3 Raising opposite arm and leg — 135
9.4 Hand-to-knee cross-patterning exercise — 136
   Variation 1 — 136
   Variation 2 — 136
9.5 Balancing pose — 137
9.6 Horizontal figure of eight — 138

■ **10. Pelvic Floor Exercise — 139**

10.1 Tensing the muscles of the pelvic floor — 141

■ **11. Exercises for the Eyes — 143**

11.1 Energizing the eyes — 145
11.2 Head and face massage — 146
11.3 Circling around a dot — 148
11.4 Watching a pendulum — 149
11.5 Exercising the eyes — 150

■ **12. Relaxation — 151**

Conscious relaxation — 152
Leading a yoga group — 154

■ **13. Exercise Guidelines — 155**

Planning a chair yoga session — 155
Fifteen-minute yoga programmes — 156
   Programme 1 — 156
   Programme 2 — 157
   Programme 3 — 157
   Programme 4 — 158

Thirty-minute yoga programmes   158

    Programme 1   158

    Programme 2 (with standing exercises)   159

    Programme 3   160

    Programme 4 (with standing exercises)   160

Forty-five-minute programmes   161

    Programme 1   161

    Programme 2   162

    Programme 3 (with standing exercises)   164

    Programme 4 (with standing exercises)   165

Sixty-minute programme   166

More About Yoga   *169*

The 'eight-fold path'   **170**

1. *Yamas* (general restrictions)   170

2. *Niyamas* (observances)   172

3. *Asana* (pose, posture)   174

4. *Pranayama* (extension of the breath/energy)   174

5. *Pratyahara* (withdrawal of the senses)   174

6. *Dharana* (concentration/composure)   175

7. *Dyana* (meditation/higher awareness)   175

8. *Samadhi* (being-at-one, ecstasy)   175

Diet   **176**

The right diet – not just for reasons of health   177

Why organic foods are preferable to those produced by conventional agricultural methods   178

Why whole foods are more nutritious and health-giving than foods made with refined flour   179

Why we should think again about eating meat   180

'Rich people's meat is poor people's hunger'   181

Sprouting seeds – green shoots from grain   181

Why sugar is harmful   182

Nuts   183

Water   184

Coffee and black tea   185

Why garlic is healthy   185

Why I Wrote this Book   *187*

INDEX   *189*

INTRODUCTION

What is chair yoga?

The history of yoga goes back more than 5000 years. It began with wise Indian hermits who studied animal behaviour, seeking to understand the secret of long life. Why does a tortoise live for 100 years or more, but a mouse only three to five years? In question was the mystery of eternal life, the fundamental pillars of which appeared to be freedom from stress, slow, deep breathing, regular exercise in fresh air, good nourishment and special methods of purification.

The wise men of India, called *rishis*, added ethical and moral rules for the human mind to this wisdom concerning the health of the body. Rectitude, non-violence and devotion to the service of mankind were a few of their fundamental principles. And so the yoga pathway came into being. The word 'yoga' is derived from '*yui*, to join', and means the union or harmony of body, mind and spirit.

Yoga has been taught for thousands of years. At first it was intended only as a way for India's spiritual elite, for the best of the best. The doctrine remained secret. But in the twentieth century, not least by means of British colonialism in India, the gateway of knowledge was opened up to the West. The first English books on yoga appeared, and in the 1940s yoga as a means to healthy living reached Germany too. In the 1960s it was popularized through the hippy movement.

In the meantime, yoga, together with Ayurveda, the science of longevity, has gained recognition as a form of bodywork, especially in the healthy living movement.

Chair yoga is relatively new. It was first developed in the 1980s by Erika Hammerström – and so yoga for the strong became yoga for the less strong. Central to this form of yoga are exercises that are suitable for people who want to do something about their health and wellbeing, but can no longer sit on a mat for hours in the lotus position, or no longer want to do headstands.

This book shows for the first time how many yoga exercises can be done sitting on a chair – exercises to activate the feet, legs, arms and hands, back, neck region, eyes and even the brain – so that those with restricted mobility no longer need give up yoga, but instead, by means of movement, can take their destiny in their hands and improve their circulation, deliver more oxygen to their cells and so gradually increase mobility and enhance brain function.

The yoga exercises that I introduce in this book can be done by almost anyone, as the approach is easy to understand and the way of doing the exercises, although much simplified, is still very effective. Whether you are old or young, whether work and/or family make heavy demands on your time or you can mostly decide for yourself how to spend your day, this kind of yoga is easy for anyone to do, as it requires no special conditions and can even be done in many everyday situations. The only genuine requirements are a chair or other means of sitting, a reasonably quiet space, indoors – or, in fine weather, outdoors – and comfortable clothing in which you can move and breathe easily.

The exercises can be done alone, at home or in a yoga group. The latter has the advantages of increasing motivation and offering the opportunity to meet new people. If you would like to learn yoga in a group, look for a teacher you like, and whose teaching appeals to you. Learning yoga in a group is more fun, and you will be keener to attend classes regularly. Avoid choosing a dogmatic teacher, for yoga has nothing to do with dogma. If you are one of those people who don't have time to attend a yoga group regularly, because your work is too demanding or you travel a lot, then this book will prompt you to practise during your journey or breaks at work. You can be flexible with this kind of yoga. Certain exercises can be done sitting on the train or aeroplane, or during a break in a car journey. Likewise, you can make tiresome waiting time at the doctor's or the bus stop more pleasant by doing a few exercises. On a seat in the park or your own garden you can make good use of the exercises, and time after work can be made more enjoyable by means of the relaxation that they bring.

The exercises in this book have been adapted in such a way that you need have no reservations about trying them, however stiff-jointed you are. The effect will be marked, and the risk of injury is slight. If you are only able to do the exercises a bit at a time, because that's the only way your body will let you, you will still have the taste of success. Yoga exercises should never be done in an acrobatic or mechanical way, but rather in a state of peace – which means a state not just of physical calm, but also of mental peace, as you enjoy spending time on an exercise. We say in yoga: a small stimulus is sufficient. Each yoga exercise should be carried out within the pain threshold, without pressure or strain.

I have structured this book in the way I run my yoga classes: we begin with extensive stretching and breathing exercises. Then we do exercises for the feet and legs, followed by ones for the hands, arms and back. Next comes the neck and shoulder region, and finally we go on to the head. To finish comes relaxation: we go through the whole body, consciously relaxing each part.

This procedure is the well-proven structure that I use in my classes, but it is by no means obligatory. All the same, you shouldn't do any exercises without first doing the stretching and breathing exercises, because conscious stretching of the whole body improves energy flow, and the breathing exercises calm your thoughts.

If you practise regularly, you will very soon feel and enjoy the effect.

■ *Why do yoga today?*

We humans have this in common: we all breathe the same air and we would like to be happy and enjoy life. The basic need to find pleasure in life presupposes a sense of wellbeing and of being at one with the things we do. Too much stress and too many problems cause lassitude, fatigue and lack of drive. Chronic stress can have this effect even on the things we actually like to do.

Yoga teaches that the place of inner peace and composure, where we can draw again and again on fresh reserves of courage and power, lies ultimately within ourselves. Of course, we can also keep looking for this state in the external world – a beautiful spot in nature, a long walk in the woods, a holiday by the sea. But which of us has time to go walking in the woods almost every day? Days off are numbered, and enough time has to be reserved for one's family or other obligations during those precious days of freedom. Therefore it's important to be able to allow regular time for rest in everyday life. Then you can learn to manage stress in a different way, and to stay calm even in trying situations.

I myself learned yoga as a young girl, at a time when I was going through a difficult phase, feeling disorientated after a six-month spell abroad. I wanted to help others, but knew that first I needed help and support myself.

Discovering yoga was a hugely important milestone in my life. At last I seemed to find the answers to many inner questions. I sensed that the yoga exercises were making me more aware and clearer in myself. I discovered more stability and composure in myself. I became more conscious of my body, and could feel more clearly whether my posture was upright as I walked, or whether my shoulders were hunching forwards because of the burden of problems I was carrying. After every yoga class I felt fresh, good humoured and well balanced, and had a different attitude to life and its challenges. I could also feel the joy of living rising in me. My social contacts became deeper, and my willingness to take risks increased.

From this time on, I practised the yoga exercises regularly. The strongest motivator for this was the wonderful sense of wellbeing during and after my hour of yoga. Just as I could feel the increased flow in my body after each exercise, so too I could go more with the flow of life. I realized that I had (and have) no influence over certain things, and stopped fretting inwardly about it. On the other hand, I began to focus on the things that I could influence in my life, and this gave me an increased sense of inner security and a new attitude to the world. It became clear to me how much my happiness lies in my own hands, and the motivation to make my life as good and beautiful as possible constantly increased. (This book is a contribution to it.)

I would like to encourage you, dear readers, to learn yoga not only for the sake of your own health, but also as a means of increasing your love of life, and your sense of refreshment and inner peace. If you feel well in your psyche, your body will also be more healthy and resilient. We would all like to be happier. Who is stopping you, apart from you yourself? Certainly, our partner is not always the person we would like them to be – likewise the children, our parents, people in authority, colleagues and friends. We can complain for the rest of our lives that people aren't the way we would like them to be – but with the help of yoga we can also learn to get along with our fellow human beings in a more understanding and loving way because, through yoga, we are practising the same way of getting along with ourselves.

All of us, nowadays, have stress aplenty, tasks that are too demanding, conflicts that seem too difficult to solve. Even children, in our society, suffer many demands, through stress at school, and fear of not being good enough and becoming an outsider. Because of the challenges we face in our achievement-orientated society, we quickly feel pushed into a corner where we keep having to struggle, often alone. Even – or perhaps especially – the people close to us challenge or provoke us over and over again. Yoga can be very helpful for enduring all these demands and finding the ability to meet them cheerfully. I myself couldn't imagine my life without yoga, quite apart from the fact that I also teach it.

If you are learning yoga, it's important not to do so in the belief that you have to have a slim and athletic body, or be a particular age, a vegetarian or a non-smoker. Simply start with the exercises and observe what happens. Just enter into that adventure. To begin with, three or five exercises are enough, but these should be done with real concentration and without external distractions. Do these exercises without a sense of pressure – and especially without a sense of pressure to succeed. Do them in the manner your body itself allows, and don't judge yourself if you don't succeed with an exercise in the way that you would like. The human body understands more quickly than you think. If you do the exercises regularly for a while, you will feel your body recalling them, and how much easier they become.

Don't force anything. Letting go and letting be are two fundamental rules for joyful yoga. If you find this difficult, practise it consciously. You will soon find that the positive value of letting go and letting be has a healing effect on your everyday life as well.

Be patient with yourself. Don't cling to the expectation of heightened body awareness straight away. This feeling comes in its own time – perhaps when you least expect it.

If you are a smoker and would like to end or reduce the habit, then do the breathing exercises very regularly for a while, once or twice a day, and just don't have the cigarette you want. Learn to let go by exhaling consciously. Do the breathing exercises, say, when you're walking in the woods as well. It may be that the desire for a cigarette will diminish more quickly than you think.

It's the same with coffee, alcohol and other drugs. Once you discover this sense of being carried and contained in yourself, your inner stability can grow and your self-awareness increases. Your perception becomes more sensitive, your sense of the essential keener, moodiness decreases. You sleep more deeply at night, and awake more refreshed. Your pleasure in life increases.

Another aspect of yoga is that it teaches the ability to be consciously in the present. Notice your own thoughts, and what you and others are saying in conversation. Many people, for much of the time, inhabit the past or the future. In today's hectic way of life, the magic of the moment is often lost. It goes unnoticed. This moment – right now – never returns just the way it is. This moment, the present, is all we really have. The past is gone, with what belongs to it, and the future is a secret – perhaps also a gift.

With regular practice of yoga and relaxation you can learn to enjoy and value the present – this very moment. I wish you much fun and pleasure in reading, and in doing the exercises.

■ *The exercises: General rules*

Don't practise yoga with a full stomach, but one hour after a light meal and about two hours after a larger one.

After each exercise, take time to feel the effect. As you do so, focus on the parts of the body that have been moving, and/or on simply breathing in and out. To begin with, you may find it difficult to concentrate solely on the breath – but this too is just a matter of practice. Gradually you'll notice that it's getting easier not to follow every thought that has nothing to do with the exercise you are doing. The more you can concentrate on your breath during the intervals for rest, the more inner peace you will feel and the more powerful will be the effect of each exercise. (And you will see that observing this is a matter of great importance.)

The exercises should be done in a well-ventilated space with an agreeable temperature. External noise should, as far as possible, be kept to a minimum.

In fine weather, I recommend doing your yoga session outdoors (albeit avoiding direct sunlight). When you have found a lovely spot in natural surroundings, you will discover the delight of relaxing to the twittering of birds, the rustling of a gentle breeze or the sound of the sea. A yoga session in the open air can be a special pleasure!

It's best not to bath, shower or swim straight after a yoga session, as yoga stimulates the flow of blood to the internal organs. Bathing, showering or swimming carries the blood back to the surface of the body, reversing the effect of the yoga exercises. Wait for an hour or two, and then you can take a bath or go for a swim.

In most of the exercises described here, there is reference to breathing. As you do each exercise, pay attention to correct inhalation and exhalation. (If, in some exercises, there is no further reference to the breath, just let it flow in and out.)

Don't answer any phone calls during your yoga session. It's best to leave the phone off the hook, or let the answering machine record the call. Interruptions would disturb the process of finding inner calm and letting go. Make sure, before you start, that you will be disturbed as little as possible. Then you will be able to relax all the more.

Make your yoga class a regular weekly event with a group where you can feel at ease and connect socially, and/or do the exercises regularly at home, as an act of self-love and self-discovery. For this, DVDs can be ordered directly from the author.

1

THE IMPORTANCE OF BREATHING PRACTICE

PRANAYAMA – *CONTROL OF THE BREATH*

Learning yoga involves, besides the physical exercises, the correct practice of breathing exercises, that is, deep, conscious, controlled breathing. Most people are shallow breathers, and don't get enough vital energy – *prana* – and oxygen to maintain a normal state of health in the nervous system and circulation. Many chronic illnesses and respiratory conditions can be prevented or relieved by correct breathing.

In yoga, correct, conscious breathing is called *pranayama*. This term is derived from Sanskrit and means 'control of the breath'. It is a compound of the words *prana* and *yama*. *Prana* means 'divine mother energy' or 'universal divine power' and *yama* means 'control' or the knowledge (or science) of control – so control of the breath is also control of energy.

Every living being is subject to this divine energy. It supports and strengthens, varies and changes, to the extent that is necessary to keep the functions of life in balance.

It is the same energy that gives us vitality and *joie de vivre* and keeps our aura cheerful and alive.

We receive most of the *prana* that we need from the air we breathe, the rest from food and water and a small proportion through our skin. *Prana* is absorbed as we breathe, through nerve endings, mainly in the nostrils. Similar nerve endings are found in the mouth and throat, and through these we absorb *prana* as we eat and drink. Therefore it's important to chew thoroughly, not only to ease digestion but in order to derive *prana* from our food. Water should always be drunk slowly, a mouthful at a time, and never with food.

Incorrect and shallow breathing leads to stiffening of the ribcage and wasting of the muscles of respiration, so that insufficient oxygen is available for healthy metabolism. In this way the cells of our body suffer incremental damage, as oxygen guarantees the complete breakdown of food into the easily eliminated end products of metabolism. If excretion of these is disturbed, the blood becomes thick and sluggish. Then the blood vessels become increasingly clogged, the heart comes under strain and blood pressure rises. Unexcreted carbon dioxide disturbs the acid–alkaline balance, and therefore exhaling correctly is just as important as inhaling correctly. Without a full out-breath, a full in-breath is impossible.

When inhalation is deep and full, blood is drawn from the periphery of the body towards the lungs, the heart fills with blood and its activity is sustained and strengthened. The coronary blood vessels receive more blood and the risk of heart disease is reduced. The activity of blood-building organs is sustained by the increased availability of oxygen.

For correct breathing it's important to breathe easily in and out, without any effort. The in-breath should take as long as the out-breath (except for some particular breathing techniques).

Clothing should be loose around the chest and abdomen, and should not restrict breathing.

Except for certain breathing exercises in which we exhale consciously through the mouth, we breathe through the nose, for this cleans the air of pathogens and dust, and warms and moistens cold air.

When doing breathing exercises, concentrate totally on the breathing process and keep consciously letting go of other thoughts.

Do the breathing exercises with the window open, or in a well-ventilated room.

Your posture should be straight or upright.

In deep, conscious breathing the shoulder girdle stays relaxed.

Correct breathing expands the lungs and makes them stronger and more resistant. It has a calming effect on the central nervous system. Emotions become more balanced. A long-term effect of conscious, deep breathing is that we breathe more deeply in the course of daily activity, and while we are asleep.

The lungs have three main lobes: the inferior, or lower abdominal (*Adham*); the middle, or thoracic (*Madhyam*); and the superior, or collar-bone, region (*Adhyam*). Breathing into the different parts, or lobes, of the lungs is the basic technique of pranayama and the beginning of good respiratory control. The three parts should first be exercised individually, and can then come seamlessly together as the single, wave-like movement of full yoga breathing.

The three lobes of the lungs are in turn divided into three segments: the front, side and back.

It's best to begin by breathing consciously into the front parts of the lungs. Later, you can breathe into the side and back parts as well.

THE BREATHING EXERCISES: MAHAT MUDRA – BREATHING INTO THE SEPARATE PARTS OF THE LUNGS

For the breathing exercises your back should be completely upright.

1.1 The inferior front part of the lungs (Adham Pranayama)

Place your hands on your abdomen, just under the bottom ribs, with the fingers together. Breathe in through your nose, slowly and freely, and slowly and freely breathe out. To begin with, it's helpful to count to three on the in-breath, and to three on the out-breath. Guide your breath consciously into your belly; feel your belly slowly rising as you breathe in, and slowly sinking as you breathe out. Feel energy and oxygen flowing into the lower part of your body and your legs.

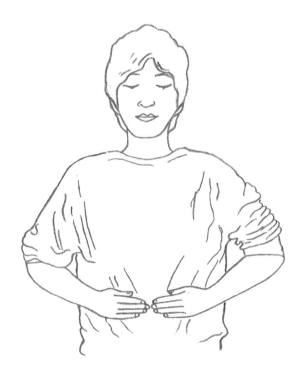

■ *1.2 The middle front part of the lungs (Madhyam Pranayama)*

After three to six breathing cycles, place your hands on your chest (keeping the fingers together the whole time, as this makes concentration easier), and count to three as you draw the breath deep into your chest. Here, too, the inhalation and exhalation should happen slowly and freely, without any effort. Feel your ribcage slowly rising and falling as you breathe, and feel the energy fizzing in your chest. This strengthens the heart muscle.

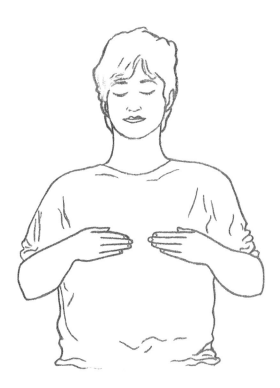

1.3 The superior front part of the lungs (Adhyam Pranayama)

After three to six breathing cycles, place your hands on your collar-bones. Feel them slightly rising as you breathe in, and slowly sinking as you breathe out. In your thoughts, guide the breath consciously upwards. The blood supply to the entire head region is increased. All the sensory organs fill with new energy, and the powers of concentration and memory are enhanced.

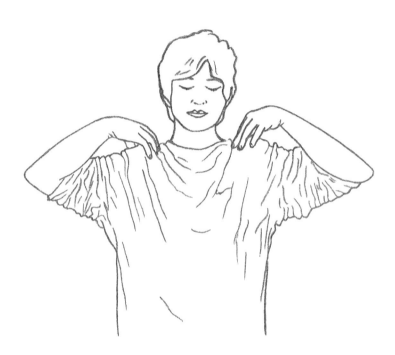

■ *1.4 Full yogic breathing (Mahat Yoga Pranayama)*

Once you feel that you can breathe into the three separate parts of the lungs, try to bring it all together.

Breathe in deeply and freely, and feel first your belly rise, then your chest, and last, your collar-bones. As you breathe out deeply and freely, first your belly sinks, then your chest and finally your collar-bones.

When you have practised this for a while, count to six on each inhalation and exhalation, twice for each part of the lungs. You can let your hands rest in your lap, or place your right hand on your abdomen and your left hand on your chest. As you inhale into the abdomen, feel your hand rising along with your belly, and as your chest lifts, feel how your left hand is lifted with it.

To feel consciously your collar-bones rising, move your right hand from your abdomen to the collar-bone area. As you exhale, move your right hand back to your belly. With your right hand feel your belly sinking, and with your left hand feel your chest sinking; and finally put your right hand back on the collar-bone area, and once again feel your collar-bones slowly sinking.

Do this wave-like inhalation and exhalation several times over again. Imagine your breath flowing very easily into you, and flowing very easily back out.

THE BREATHING EXERCISES: BREATHING INTO THE SIDE AND BACK PARTS OF THE LUNGS

1.5 The lower side and back region of the lungs

Place your hands at your waist and direct the breath consciously into the lower side region of both lungs. Imagine that you are breathing into your hands. After three to six breath cycles (initially), place your hands on your back, at waist level. Take care, with your hands in this position, that the thumbs are not extended out to the sides but are alongside your fingers, in contact with your back. Now direct your breath consciously into the lower back region of your lungs. Again, imagine breathing into your hands. This may be difficult to begin with, but imagining it will help you. After three to six breathing cycles, let your hands drop into your lap and notice what you are feeling.

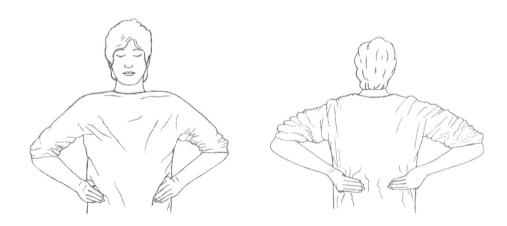

■ 1.6 The middle part of the side and back region of the lungs

Lay both hands on the sides of your chest. Direct your breath deep into the places under your hands. After three to six breathing cycles, place your hands as best you can on the middle of your back and direct your breath there for three to six breathing cycles.

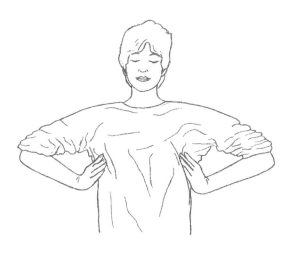

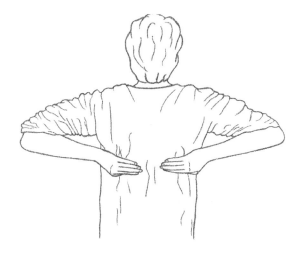

■ 1.7 The upper side and back region of the lungs

Now place your hands on either side of your waist and guide your breath consciously into your armpits. Breathe consciously into the upper side region of your lungs. After three to six breathing cycles, place your hands on your upper back and breathe consciously into the upper back region of your lungs. To begin with, you may find it difficult to imagine that you can breathe specifically into these areas – but, in fact, you can, and with regular practice you will keep improving.

Then gradually increase the number of breathing cycles to nine and more. Allow an equal amount of time for breathing into each region of your lungs. Then notice how you are feeling and enjoy the calming, balancing effect on your thoughts and feelings.

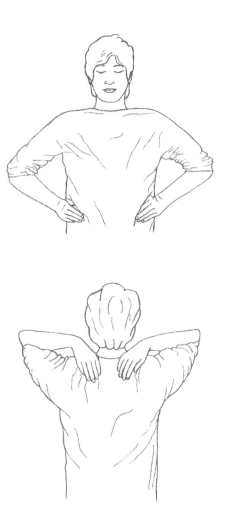

■ *1.8* Savitri Pranayama

Savitri is the name of the goddess of the sun and the seasons. This breathing exercise consists of a four-part breathing rhythm: inhale, hold the breath, exhale, pause breathing. The rhythm linked to these four functions is 2–1–2–1. As a beginner, count:

- ■ *two* as you breathe in

- ■ *one* as you hold your breath

- ■ *two* as you exhale

- ■ *one* as you pause breathing.

Breathe for a series of at least nine cycles. For this exercise you can lean comfortably against the backrest of your chair, but take care to have your back upright and your shoulders relaxed. Or practise this breathing rhythm lying down, when you may find that you can relax even better. Make sure that your body is pleasantly warm, covered up if need be. In lying down, these breathing rhythms bring the body rest; in sitting, renewed strength and energy.

You can carry out the following breathing rhythms for up to 20 minutes, for optimal effect. Begin with the shortest sequence, for at least nine cycles. The next time, increase the number of cycles. When you can do the shortest sequence without difficulty, try the next one, and later the next, for nine cycles; increase the number on each successive occasion. Regular, daily practice is especially effective. Counting the rhythms should be done slowly, with concentration.

The effect of Savitri Pranayama

BREATHING RHYTHM 4–2–4–2
Supports convalescence following illness; suitable for children who are interested in yoga.

BREATHING RHYTHM 6–3–6–3

Helps with sleep disturbance; has a soothing effect. Helpful for depression and other nervous and psychosomatic conditions.

BREATHING RHYTHM 8–4–8–4

Supports the formation of cells, bones and marrow, muscles and blood; stimulates the lymphatic system.

1.9 Alternate nostril breathing (Surya Bhedana Pranayama)

Sit up comfortably, with your back straight and your shoulders relaxed. It is advisable for beginners to do this exercise in front of a mirror, in order to check that your posture remains erect while you are doing it.

- Raise your right hand and close your left nostril with your fourth finger.

- Inhale slowly and deeply through the right nostril.

- Now, with your thumb, close the right nostril and exhale slowly and deeply through the left nostril.

- Now inhale through the left nostril again, slowly and deeply; once more close the left nostril with your fourth finger and exhale through the right nostril, slowly and deeply.

- Now inhale again slowly through the right nostril; close it again with your thumb, and exhale slowly through the left nostril.

Repeat this exercise for at least nine cycles. Beginning by inhaling through the right nostril, and end by exhaling through the left nostril.

Take care that your upper body and head remain erect, with your shoulders and right arm relaxed.

When you have mastered this breathing exercise, you can combine it with a *Savitri* breathing rhythm (see previous exercise).

- As you inhale through the right nostril, count to four.

- Close the right nostril and count to two.

- As you exhale through the left nostril, count to four.

- Pause breathing and count to two.

- Inhale again through the left nostril, count to four.

- Close the left nostril, count to two.

- Exhale through the right nostril, count to four, etc.

When you can manage the 4–2–4–2 rhythm well, you can gradually advance to the longer counts.

Effect

This exercise helps with insomnia, calms mental and emotional turmoil, purifies the blood, soothes headaches and is supportive for anxious and depressive conditions. Much recommended at the end of a taxing day at work, when you are tired, weary and not in a mood to relax because you can't let go of so many thoughts. Alternate nostril breathing has a profoundly calming effect.

2

EXERCISES FOR THE FEET AND TOES

The feet are the roots of the body. If they are supple and springy they can withstand physical shocks, and in this way protect the spine. Stiff feet, with every step, send a harsh impact rippling up into the knees, hips and back, causing wear of the joints and vertebrae. So well-trained foot muscles have an important part to play in our wellbeing.

Also, reflex zones for the entire body are located in the feet – so a foot massage is always relaxing and helps to maintain the back and the digestive system.

So let's begin at the roots and allow our feet to regain contact with the earth, in the same way as a wild vine attaches itself to the wall of a house.

Before you start the foot exercises, please take time to become really aware of your feet:

- Which parts of your feet are touching the ground?

- Which are the weight-bearing parts?

- What changes in your foot when you bend your toes like claws?

- How does it feel if you gently shift or rock your body?

Then take a few breaths through your nose; imagine that the breath is flowing right down into the soles of your feet, and back out of your body through your nose.

Now that you have arrived in your feet, you can begin the exercises.

The foot exercises are beneficial in many ways: they activate the musculature of the feet, restore mobility to the toes and ankles and ensure warmth and good circulation to the feet – and in so doing they contribute to a general state of wellbeing. Some of these exercises can even be done in bed, before you get up in the morning.

For the following exercises, sit near enough to the edge of your chair for the soles of your feet to be in full contact with the floor. Your feet and knees should be about shoulder-width apart, in a stable triangle in relation to your bottom. Your spine is erect and your head, back and pelvis are aligned with one another. Your shoulders are relaxed and your hands are loose as they rest on your thighs.

2.1 Raising the heels

Have your feet at right angles to your knees, so that the calves are like two pillars supporting the knees. Now lift your right and left heels alternately. Do this about ten times. Send your awareness keenly into the bones as your foot rolls over them. Remember to let your breath flow normally.

Effect

This exercise stimulates blood flow to the feet and calves, prevents varicose veins and eases problems caused by them. Via the reflex zones in the feet it relaxes the whole spine and is helpful for all kinds of back problems.

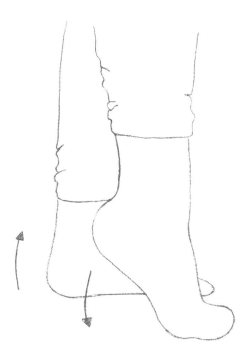

■ 2.2 Rocking on the soles of the feet

Alternately raise first the toes and then the heels of both feet, resulting in a rocking movement. Do this five to ten times. Let your breath flow.

Effect

This exercise stimulates circulation to the feet and calves, prevents varicose veins and eases problems associated with them.

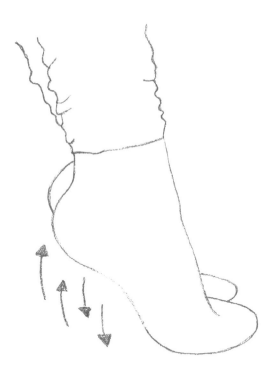

■ *2.3 Rolling the feet*

Place your feet shoulder-width apart. Roll your feet inwards and outwards a few times, so that the inner and outer edges of your feet meet the floor alternately.

Effect

This exercise loosens the musculature of the feet and relaxes the foot and hip joints.

For the following exercises you can rest comfortably, but upright, against the back of your chair.

■ 2.4 *Waking up the feet*

Move your feet to and fro, slightly clenching the toes and the soles, and then stretching them out again. Do this to-and-fro movement several times.

Effect

This exercise keeps the feet and toes supple, and, via the reflex zones, works on the shoulder girdle, the neck region of the spine, the eyes and the ears.

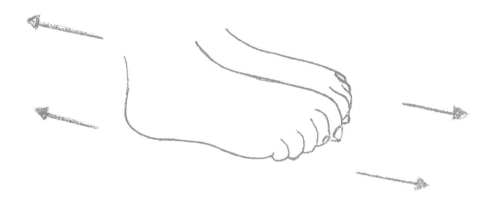

2.5 Loosening and spreading the toes

Raise your right foot. Loosen the toes and spread them out, three times. Do the same with your left foot.

Effect

Maintains or improves the suppleness of the foot, and activates the muscles of the legs and back.

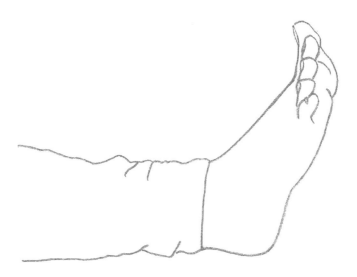

2.6 Clenching the toes

Raise your right foot and draw the toes towards you. Feel the stretch through the sole of your foot. Now clench your toes. Feel the wrinkling in the sole. Stretch and clench your toes three times. Let the foot sink back down. Repeat the exercise with your left foot. Breathe quietly as you do this.

Effect

This exercise keeps the toes supple and improves circulation, eases tension in the toes and stimulates the reflex zones in the feet.

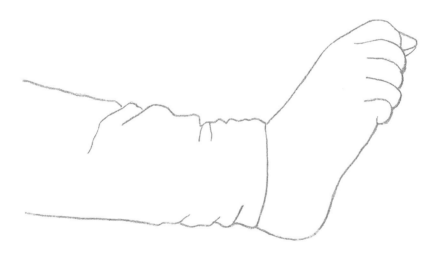

■ *2.7 Stretching the feet*

Raise your right foot. As you inhale, bring the whole foot towards you; and as you exhale, stretch it away. Do this three times, slowly and with awareness. Then circle your foot from the ankle, several times to the right, and then to the left. Let your right foot drop. Repeat the exercise with your left foot.

Variation

Raise both feet slightly and stretch them both together, alternately upwards and downwards; do this several times. Then move your feet a little bit apart and circle from the ankles, to the right and to the left, or inwards and outwards. Let your breath flow gently as you do this.

Effect

This exercise stimulates circulation to the feet, ankles and calves. It helps keep the ankles supple.

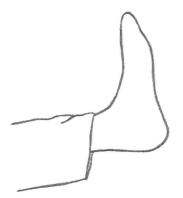 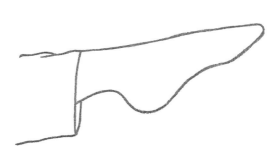

■ 2.8 Walking on tiptoe and on the heels

Stand up and take a few steps on tiptoe, then on your heels, then again on tiptoe, and again on your heels. Repeat several times.

Effect

This exercise strengthens the foot muscles and the toes.

3

EXERCISES FOR THE LEGS

The legs are the pillars of the body and, like the pillars of a Greek temple, they carry their load best if the pillars are the same distance apart as the width of the body resting on them: hip-width apart.

Just see how it feels when your legs are close together and your feet touching. How easy it would be for someone to topple you over! A breath of wind would do it.

Now stand with your legs hip-width apart. Feel how easy standing is, like this. No one could knock you off balance in a hurry.

Feel into your legs. Are they parallel, or do they bend inwards or outwards?

How do they feel – light, would you say, or heavy?

If you have varicose vein problems it's a good idea to put your feet up for 15 minutes at least once a day, so that the venous blood doesn't pool, but flows back to the heart. While blood is pushed through the arteries by the heart, the most powerful pump in the body, it has to make its own way back. The veins have little valves that prevent it from flowing backwards, but they have no pump of their own, so they depend on the movement of muscles surrounding them. So good leg muscles don't just help the veins, they take pressure off the heart as well.

The exercises in this chapter bring many benefits: they stimulate lubrication of the knee joints by means of movement without weight-bearing, improve circulation and cleanse tissue, and activate veins, the lymphatic system and digestion.

■ 3.1 Pushing the knees sideways

With your knees shoulder-width apart, place your hands on the inside of both knees. On the next inhalation try to press your knees together, while pressing hard the opposite way with your hands. Briefly hold the tension. As you exhale, let go, loosen up. Repeat the exercise three times.

Now put your hands on the outside of your knees. As you inhale, try to push your knees apart, again pressing hard against them with your hands. Briefly hold the tension…and let go as you exhale. Do this exercise three times and to finish, shake your legs. Then you can bring your hands back into your lap and feel into your legs.

Effect

The exercise strengthens the leg muscles and the muscles that stabilize the hips.

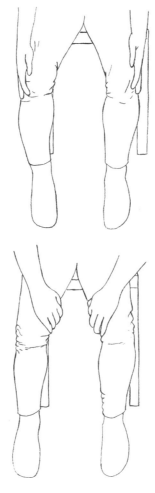

■ 3.2 Massaging the legs

Rub first your knees, then the backs of your knees and your calves. Then rub firmly over your thighs and hips, and gently over the kidney area (in the small of your back). Now rest your hands in your lap and feel into the parts that you have massaged.

Effect

The exercise stimulates circulation to the legs, hip joints and kidney area. It supports the bladder and kidneys, as the bladder and kidney meridian runs through the knees.

■ 3.3 Bending the legs

Sit on the front of your chair. Stretch out your right leg, link both hands behind the right knee, straighten your back and inhale. As you exhale, slowly bend your right knee and let your head sink towards it – or you can briefly touch your knee with your nose. Then, as you inhale, sit up straight and stretch your leg out again. As you exhale, bend your knee again and drop your head. Repeat this one more time. Then lower your right leg, notice how it feels…and repeat the exercise with your left leg.

Effect

This exercise keeps the knee and hip joints resilient, stimulates the intestines, cleanses the liver, gallbladder and pancreas, and eases bloating and tension in the abdominal region.

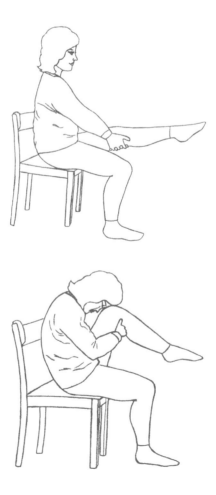

■ 3.4 Making circles with the heels

Slide your bottom a little way forwards, but keep your back supported by the chair. Raise your right leg and make circles with your right heel – small ones to begin with, then gradually make them larger. Then circle in the opposite direction, gradually making the circles smaller again. Lower your right foot slowly and feel into your right leg and right hip. Then make circles with your left heel. As you do so, breathe deeply and evenly into your abdomen.

Effect

This exercise strengthens the leg muscles and keeps the hip joints supple.

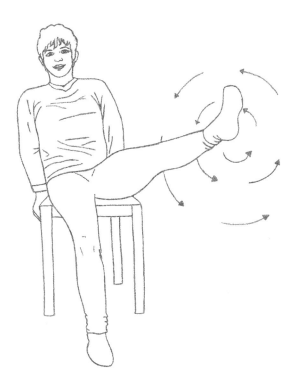

■ 3.5 *Wind-releasing exercise* (Pavanmuktasana)

For this exercise, again, sit a bit further forwards on your chair.

■ Stretch your left leg out gently, with the sole of the left foot touching the floor. As you inhale, bend your right leg. Place both hands around the right knee.

■ As you exhale, press your right thigh gently against your belly and drop your head.

■ In this position inhale a bit more deeply and hold your breath, and the position, for one or two seconds.

■ As you exhale, let out the breath with a hiss, lower your right leg and raise your head, so that you are sitting upright again.

Do this exercise three times with your right leg, and three times with the left. After a short pause to feel the effect, bend both knees as you inhale; do this too – if it's not too difficult – three times. Then lean over forwards and let go. Finally sit up again, rest against the back of your chair and enjoy noticing what you are feeling.

Effect

This exercise helps with bloating. It releases tension and gives the internal organs a bit of acupressure.

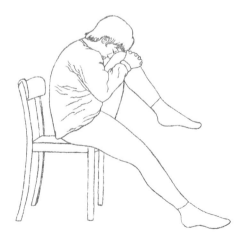

■ 3.6 Clapping under the legs

Lift your legs alternately, and each time clap your hands under the raised leg. Do this 10–15 times, alternating the legs. Then relax for a little while.

Effect

This exercise stimulates the circulation and invigorates you.

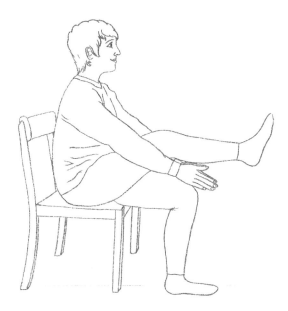

■ 3.7 Bicycling

For this exercise you can slide your bottom forwards and lean back against the chair. Raise your right leg and 'pedal' a few revolutions forwards and then backwards – five to seven times each way. Lower your right leg and feel into it. Do the same with your left leg.

Variation for advanced students with good abdominal muscles

After a brief interval, and if it's not too strenuous, pedal as if you were sitting on a bicycle, or – even more difficult – pedal with both legs in the same direction, several revolutions forwards, and then backwards. Then lower your legs slowly and lean forward, dangling your arms. Sit up again, rest against the back of the chair, and feel into your legs and abdomen. Notice the improved energy flow and stimulation of circulation. If you feel the need, inhale once or twice deeply through your nose, and exhale through your mouth, with a sigh. This relieves pressure on the heart.

Effect

This exercise strengthens the muscles of the legs and abdomen, and stimulates circulation.

Be careful: The 'advanced' variation requires well-developed abdominal muscles – otherwise it can have a negative impact on the back.

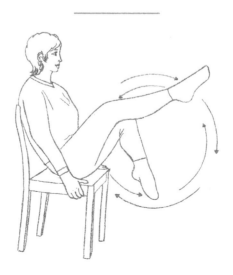

■ 3.8 Stimulating lymph flow in the lower part of the body

- ■ Sit on the front of your chair, with your body upright.

- ■ Push your left leg a little way out in front of you, with the sole of your left foot staying in contact with the floor.

- ■ Bend your right leg and place your hands around your right knee.

- ■ As you inhale, press your right thigh gently towards your belly; as you exhale, let go a little, so that your thigh moves slightly away from your belly. (Your hands remain in position around your knee.)

- ■ Repeat these movements a few times, in coordination with your breathing – slowly, five to seven times.

- ■ On an exhalation release your hands and slowly lower your leg.

Now, with your hands resting in your lap, feel into the right side of your lower back and the right side of your abdomen. Then follow the same procedure with your left leg.

Variation for advanced students with good abdominal muscles

- ■ After a short pause to feel into your lower back and abdomen on the left side, draw both knees towards you – as long as this is not too difficult for you.

- ■ Place your hands around your knees and move both thighs several times, in time with your breathing.

- ■ After five to seven times, lower your legs again slowly. Then raise energy into your hands by rubbing the palms together vigorously.

- ■ Place your hands on your lower back, over the place where the lymph nodes are. Leave your hands there for a few seconds.

■ For a second and third time, rub your hands and place them over your lower back.

■ Lean back against the chair, and once again feel into your lower back and abdomen. Consciously enjoy the experience of what you are feeling.

Effect

This exercise stimulates lymph flow in the lower part of the body. The lymph nodes are energetically stimulated and supported. The abdominal organs are massaged and receive gentle acupressure.

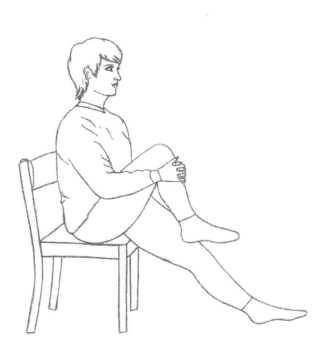

■ *3.9 Boat pose*

Variation 1 (*Navasana*)

Stretch your legs and arms (as far as possible together, all at once) out in front of you. Briefly hold the stretch, and your breath. As you exhale, slowly lower your arms and legs. Repeat the exercise – and twice more, if it's not too difficult. The third time, stay in the stretch and let your breathing flow.

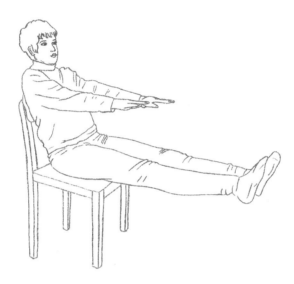

Variation 2 (*Nava Kriya*)

As you inhale, stretch your legs out in front again, make fists with your hands and circle vigorously with your arms, holding your breath as you do so. Exhale, sighing loudly through your mouth, and lower your legs and arms; lean forwards and let go completely. Repeat twice.

Effect

The energy that was gathered into the middle of the body in Variation 1 is distributed into the trunk in Variation 2 in such a way that the body can release stale energy. Both variations strengthen the muscles of the abdomen, legs and arms. Variation 2, in addition, stimulates circulation and releases tension.

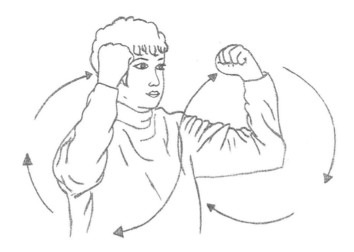

4

EXERCISES FOR THE FINGERS, HANDS AND WRISTS

We realize how important our hands are only when we are unable to use them. We need them for getting dressed, eating – indeed, for the smallest of actions. It was manual dexterity that turned humans into craftsmen, and made our development from animal to human possible. We give small children things to feel with their hands, because manual dexterity goes together with the development of the brain.

Take time to have a good look at your hands. They tell a story – the story of your work. A farmer's hands are calloused and powerful, from gripping and handling. A dancer's hands are elegant and well manicured.

Someone's hands might be always red, sweaty and warm…or maybe they are frequently cold and bluish? So hands also tell you about blood pressure and the condition of blood vessels.

When was the last time you spent time on your hands, which work so well for you every day? Feel into your hands. Can you move each finger individually?

Can you feel into each fingertip?

Does the little finger feel different from the thumb?

Turn the palms of your hands first towards the earth, and then towards the sky. Can you feel the difference?

The benefits of the hand exercises in this book are many and varied: they make the fingers supple and strong, promote good circulation and warm the hands, and strengthen the muscles of the arms and the flow of lymph, even in the chest.

These exercises are especially important for anyone with gout or rheumatism. Movement promotes efficient removal of waste products from tissues, and stretches shortened tendons.

4.1 Interlacing the fingers (an exercise to develop skill)

- Stretch your arms out in front of you. Then cross your right hand over the left one.

- Bring the palms of your hands together and lace your fingers.

- Rotate the two hands in a semicircle, downwards and up towards your chest – your hands should not touch your chest.

- Then, if you can, raise and lower each finger separately. For example, raise your ring finger and then lower it again. You can choose which sequence to follow.

- Then separate your hands and loosen them up.

Effect

This exercise keeps the fingers and wrists supple and coordinates and integrates the two hemispheres of the brain.

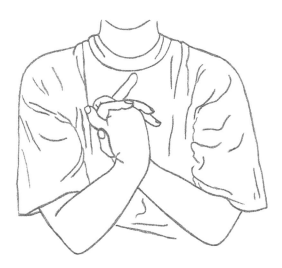

■ 4.2 *Pressing the fingertips together*

Bring your fingertips together. As you inhale, press your arms and hands against each other, and as you exhale, release the pressure. Then repeat the exercise more quickly and a bit jerkily, so that you feel the effect of pressing your arms together in the muscles of your chest as well. Do this, rapidly, 15–20 times. Shake out your hands and feel the difference.

Effect

This exercise strengthens the chest muscles, keeps the bust in good shape, strengthens the muscles of the arms, hands and fingers, and activates lymph in the chest (prophylactic for breast cancer).

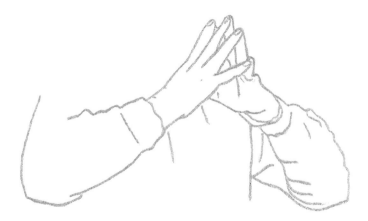

■ 4.3 Locking the fingers together

Lock the fingers of both hands together. On the next inhalation pull your arms away from one another; as you exhale, relax them again. (Keep your fingers locked the whole time.) Repeat the exercise three times. Then separate your fingers and shake out your arms and hands.

Effect

This exercise strengthens the muscles of the arms, hands and fingers, and activates lymph in the chest.

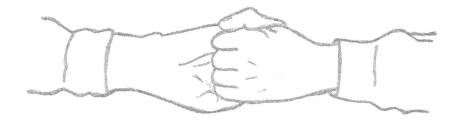

■ 4.4 Pressing the palms of the hands together

Place the palms of your hands together. As you inhale, press your hands together hard; as you exhale, release them. Repeat the exercise three times. Then shake out your hands, or go straight on to the next exercise.

Effect

This exercise strengthens the muscles of the arms and hands, and activates lymph in the chest.

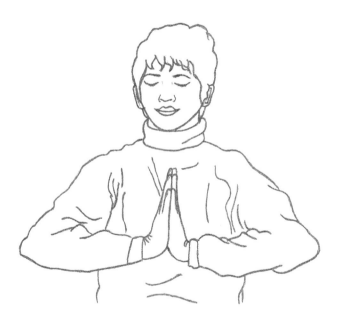

■ 4.5 Moving all the fingers separately

Take your hands up and out to the sides, with the elbows bent, and spread your fingers wide apart. Then press your thumbs against the palms of your hands, and hold for two seconds. Extend your thumbs. Then press your index fingers against the palms of your hands, and hold for a moment. Do the same with the middle, ring and little fingers. Then you can repeat the sequence in reverse.

Effect

This exercise keeps the fingers supple, stimulates circulation in the fingers and hands, loosens stiff fingers and prevents pain in the finger joints.

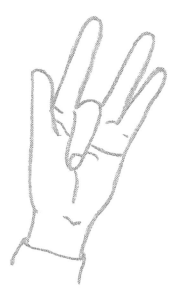

■ 4.6 *Making circles with the fingers*

Take your hands out to the sides and up to chest or shoulder height. Now make a few circles with both thumbs, then a few with your index fingers, then your middle and ring fingers. When you get to your little fingers, circle first in one direction and then in the other.

Then circle your ring fingers in the new direction, and the same for your middle and index fingers and your thumbs.

Shake out your hands and arms and feel into your fingers.

Effect

This exercise keeps the fingers and finger joints supple.

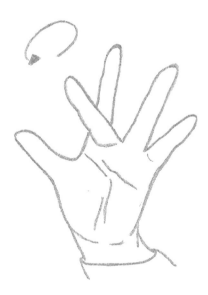

4.7 Fingertips touching

As in the previous exercise, take your hands upwards and out to the sides. Bring the index finger and thumb of each hand together, then the middle finger and thumb, the ring finger and thumb, and the little finger and thumb. Then repeat the sequence in reverse, beginning with the little finger and finishing with the index finger. You might also do the exercise a bit more quickly.

Effect

This exercise increases the power of concentration and keeps the fingers supple.

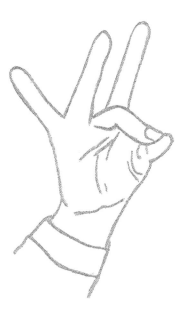

■ 4.8 Spreading out the fingers / making fists

Stretch out your arms in front of you. As you inhale, make fists; as you exhale, spread out your fingers. Do this three to six times.

Then keep your hands in fists. Circle your fists from the wrists, first inwards, then outwards.

Effect

This exercise strengthens the wrists and the arm muscles, and stimulates circulation in the veins.

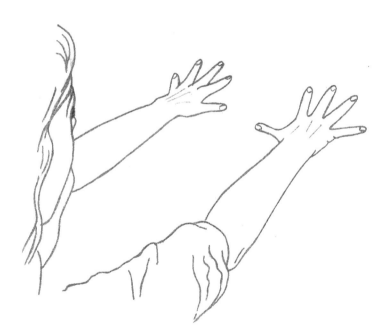

■ *4.9 Opening the hands*

For this exercise sit with your back straight, resting against the back of your chair.

Place your hands in the prayer position in front of your chest. The elbows are level with the wrists. On the next inhalation, push your elbows backwards, so that your hands open out and forwards. As you exhale, bring the palms of your hands back together, so that they are touching again. You can do this exercise three to five times, slowly and in a meditative way.

Effect

The exercise has a harmonizing effect on the entire chest region.

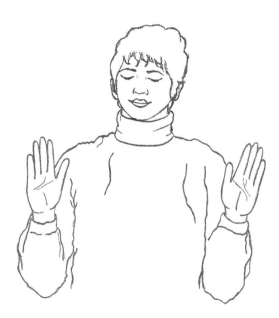

■ *4.10 The bud*

Make tight fists with your hands. Imagine that your fists are two flowers slowly opening in the sun. With strong pressure, slowly open your hands and spread out your fingers until they are wide open. Hold the tension briefly. Then close your hands slowly, with equal, opposite pressure, back into fists. Loosen your hands and fingers. Repeat once or twice more.

Effect

This exercise keeps the fingers supple, stimulates circulation in the hands and fingers, loosens stiff fingers, prevents pain in the finger joints, stretches tendons and harmonizes the hand meridians.

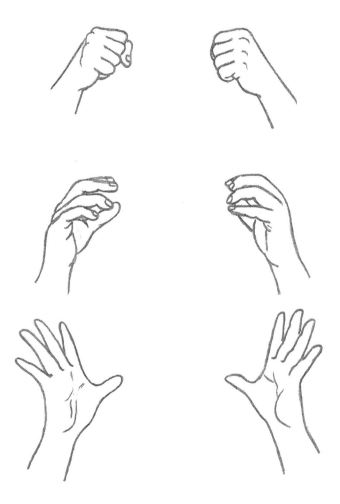

■ *4.11 Exercise for the wrists*

Stretch out your arms in front, so that the palms are directed forwards and the fingertips pointing upwards. As you inhale, turn your hands inwards, so that (ideally) the fingertips are aligned; as you exhale, turn your hands outwards. Your arms should be stretched out the whole time. Repeat this exercise three to six times. Then relax your arms and let them drop into your lap.

Effect

This exercise keeps the wrists supple and strengthens them, as well as the muscles of the arms, and harmonizes the arm meridians.

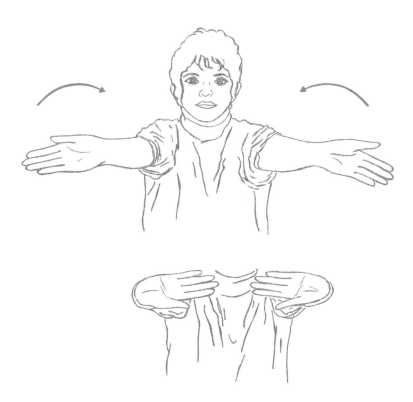

■ 4.12 Bending the wrists

Stretch out your arms in front, with the palms facing downwards. Now, as you inhale, bend your hands upwards from the wrists; as you exhale, bend your hands downwards from the wrists. Repeat three to five times. The arms remain stretched out the whole time.

Effect

This exercise strengthens the wrists and underarm muscles, and harmonizes the arm meridians.

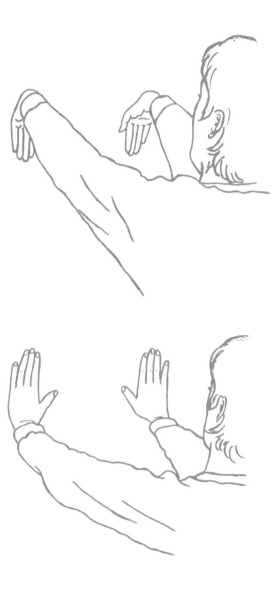

■ *4.13 Stretching the hands*

Raise your hands to shoulder height, with arms bent at the elbows. As you inhale, let your hands drop backwards, with the palms facing upwards. (The fingers are relaxed and slightly bent.) As you exhale, let your hands drop forwards, so that now the palms are facing downwards.

Effect

This exercise strengthens the wrists.

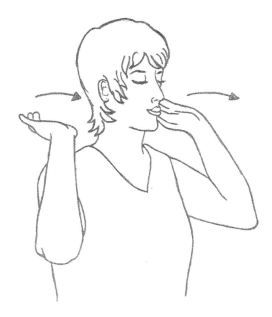

Variation

This exercise can also be done with the fingers spread out.

Effect

In either variation the underarm muscles are also stretched and strengthened, short tendons are stretched and the hand meridians harmonized.

5

EXERCISES FOR THE ARMS

Our arms are like the branches of the tree. Their movement has a harmonizing effect on the trunk. The trunk of our body-tree consists of the spine, back, pelvis, abdomen, thorax and shoulder joints. The arms, then, should not hang limp and 'sapless' by the sides of the body, but should possess a particular lively tone. With a bit of training the arm muscles will take the strain off the wrists, elbows, shoulders and even the neck. Imagine a heavy shopping bag hanging from your hands and dragging your arms down, straining your wrists to the limit and drying them out. If, instead, your muscles (and not your bones) are carrying the bag, then the joints stay intact and 'juicy'. This doesn't mean doing 'bodybuilding' with heavy weights – but rather light, gentle training that supplies the muscles with fresh blood and oxygen, and in this way encourages them to grow.

Feel into your arms. How do they feel? Are they limp rubber bands, gnarled branches or supple young willow wands?

Raise one arm and feel the increase in venous blood flowing back to the heart. Lower your arm again. Can you feel the difference, compared to the arm that you haven't moved?

Swing both arms to and fro. Can you feel how the swing livens up your body? Can you feel your back loosening up?

Stop, and feel once more into your arms. Can you feel the blood pulsing?

Arm exercises bring many benefits: they stimulate circulation, and thereby the heart and lungs, activate the flow of lymph in the chest, loosen up the back, make the shoulders supple, ease tension in the shoulders and neck, strengthen the arm muscles, widen the thorax, creating more breathing space, and enhance the supply of oxygen to the brain.

Be careful: As with all other exercises – don't overdo it. Start with a few easy exercises and build up slowly. The body should have fun with yoga, look forward to new energy and not feel overtaxed. If you get stiff muscles, then you have over-exercised and not breathed enough. Take better care of yourself, observe what does you good, and to what degree.

■ *5.1 Making circles with the arms*

Variation 1

■ Sit on the front of your chair and place the palm of your left hand on the middle of your chest.

■ Now move your right arm in a circle, forwards five times and backwards five times. Breathe normally as you do this.

■ Then lower your hands onto your thighs and feel into your right shoulder and arm.

■ Now place your right palm on the middle of your chest and make circles with your left arm, backwards and then forwards.

■ Then lean over forwards and let your arms dangle loosely.

Effect

This exercise stimulates the flow of energy and blood to the heart and lungs, keeps the shoulder joints supple, activates the arm meridians and the flow of lymph in the chest, and harmonizes the thoracic spine.

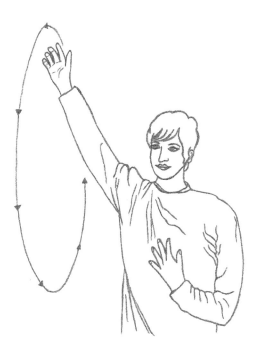

Variation 2

For this variation on circles with the arms you can rest comfortably, but upright, against the back of your chair. Look into the palm of your right hand – the thumb is stretched out. As you inhale, raise your arm out in front of you, make a circle upwards and, as you exhale, continue in a backwards direction to complete the circle. Make a circle three times, slowly and deliberately, all the time looking into the palm of your hand. Then do the same exercise three times with your left arm.

These arm circles should be carried out much more slowly than those in Variation 1.

Effect

This exercise is good for the eyes and keeps the shoulder joints supple.

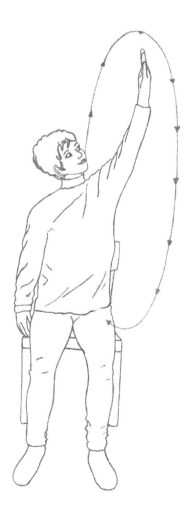

5.2 Extending the elbows

Raise your elbows to shoulder height by your sides, with your fingers pointing towards each other and lightly touching. As you inhale, extend your shoulders and elbows slowly out and back (keeping your hands and upper arms in the same alignment); as you exhale, bring your arms forwards again, so that the fingertips meet. Repeat once or twice. The last time, hold the backwards extension for a few seconds and let your breath flow. When you have completed the exercise, lower your arms slowly. Loosen your hands and arms. Feel consciously into your shoulders and upper back. Let the exercise continue to take effect during a break for rest.

Effect

This exercise loosens the shoulder and neck region and the upper back, eases tension and strengthens the muscles of the upper back, shoulders and chest.

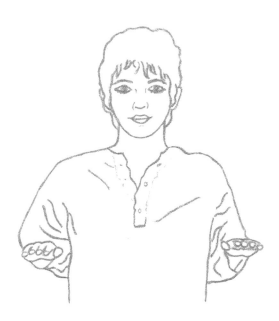

■ *5.3 Widening the chest*

■ Sit on the front edge of your chair.

■ Make fists with your hands and raise your arms to chest height. Inhale.

■ As you exhale, open your arms wide (still with fists), so that your chest widens.

■ As you inhale, bring your arms back to chest height; as you exhale, open your arms out to the sides again and feel really powerful as you do so.

■ Repeat this exercise two or three times.

■ Lower your hands into your lap and enjoy the after-effect.

Effect

This exercise strengthens the lungs, as the lung meridian is stretched. It also strengthens the muscles of the arms, eases tensions in the shoulders and improves attention to the breath and concentration.

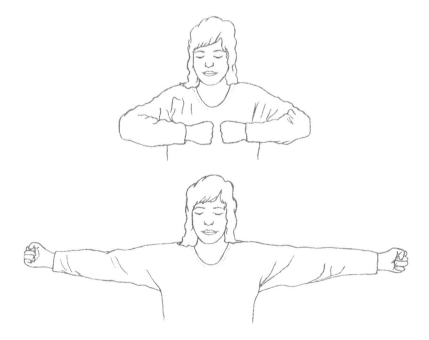

■ 5.4 Relaxing the ribcage

■ Bend your arms at waist level; the upper arms stay close to your body.

■ Stretch your forearms out in front, with the palms of your hands upwards.

■ On the next exhalation turn your forearms slowly outwards – only as far as the pain threshold – and let your chin sink onto your breastbone.

■ As you inhale, raise your head again and bring your arms back to the starting position.

■ Repeat this exercise three or four times.

Effect

This exercise expands the muscles of the chest and improves the shape of the chest; it opens the ribcage, stimulates chest lymph and eases shoulder tension.

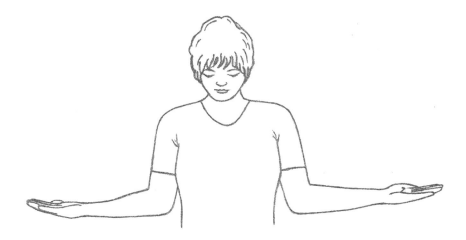

■ 5.5 *Crossing your arms*

Open out your arms and raise them to shoulder height, with the palms facing inwards and the fingers together. As you inhale, lift your outstretched arms up higher in an easy semicircular movement, so that your hands cross above your head. As you exhale, lower your arms back down to shoulder level. Repeat twice.

Effect

This exercise strengthens the shoulder joints and the lateral musculature of the trunk, opens out the intercostal musculature and creates more breathing space. It improves upper chest breathing to give enhanced oxygen supply to the brain.

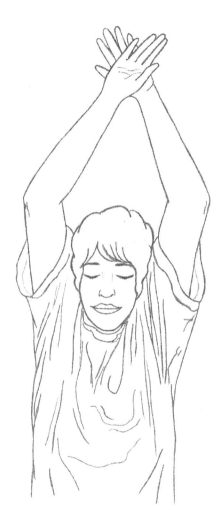

5.6 Stretching the arms

Clasp your hands together at chest height, interlacing your fingers. As you inhale, draw the palms of your hands towards your chest; as you exhale, stretch the palms away from you. Repeat three to five times.

Effect

The arm muscles are stretched, the arm meridians harmonized, and overall this exercise has a calming effect.

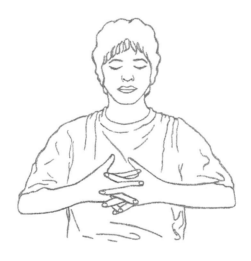

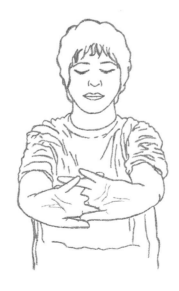

■ 5.7 *Harmonizing exercise*

Important for this exercise is the correct position of the hands and arms: the elbows should be in line with the wrists, the palms together. This old Asiatic prayer posture is called *Namaskara Mudra*.

■ Lean against the back of your chair.

■ Bring your hands into the prayer position in front of your chest.

■ As you inhale, stretch your arms out in front of you (with the palms directed forwards); as you exhale, lengthen your arms down to your sides.

■ On the next inhalation fold your hands above your head, and as you exhale, stretch your hands upwards (with the palms toward the ceiling).

■ As you breathe in, release your hands, lower your arms slowly outwards to your sides; as you breathe out, bring your hands back together in the prayer position in front of your chest.

■ Repeat twice more.

Effect

This exercise has a harmonizing effect, calms the nerves and senses, and strengthens chest breathing and the heart.

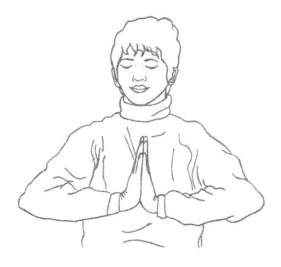

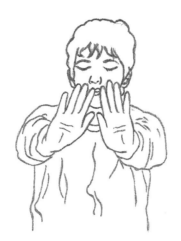

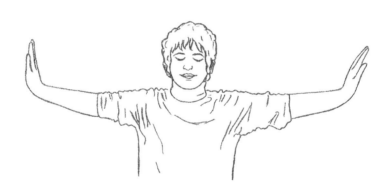

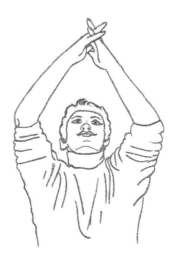

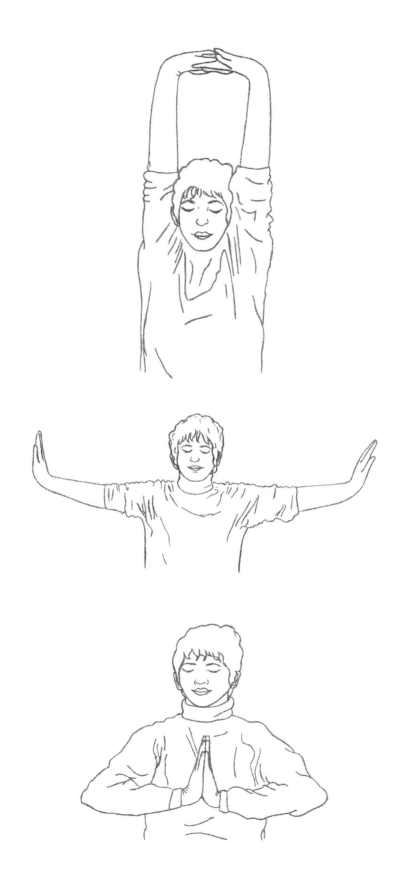

■ 5.8 'PAH' exercise – loosening up the arms

Place your hands with the palms against your collar-bones. Inhale deeply. With a loud 'PAH' thrust your hands away from you and let go of all tension in your arms. Do this exercise five to seven times, and imagine that you are flinging away anything that threatens you. It is very important to say 'PAH' out loud as you do this, so that inner tensions are voiced and thereby more intensely expressed.

Effect

This exercise releases inner tension and relaxes the muscles of the arms, mobilizes the spine and gives flexibility in the vital axis.

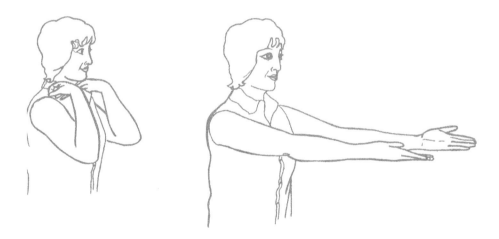

■ *5.9 Mountain pose – upward stretch*

Variation 1

- ■ Sit at the front of your chair.

- ■ As you inhale, slowly raise your arms sideways and stretch them up over your head until the palms of your hands meet. Hold the stretch, and your breath, for a little while.

- ■ As you exhale, slowly lower your arms back down by your sides and into your lap.

- ■ Do this stretch three times. The third time, stay in the stretch for three to five breaths and let your breath flow.

- ■ As you exhale, lower your arms back down by your sides, bend over forwards and briefly let your arms dangle.

- ■ Slowly sit up with your upper body erect, and feel the effect.

Effect

This exercise lengthens the spine, strengthens the lungs and eases tension in the upper back and the neck and shoulder region.

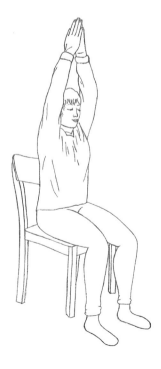

Variation 2

■ Place your right hand on your right shoulder, and your left hand on your left shoulder. Your back should be straight.

■ As you inhale, stretch your arms upwards, so that the palms of your hands are facing each other; briefly hold the stretch, and your breath.

■ As you exhale, slowly lower your hands back down onto your shoulders.

■ Do this three times. The third time, stay in the upward stretch, let your breathing flow and pump (alternately making fists and then spreading out your fingers) a few times vigorously with your hands.

■ After three to nine breathing cycles slowly lower your arms. Lean over forwards, let go completely and dangle.

■ Sit up again slowly and feel consciously into your upper back.

Effect

This exercise lengthens the spine, strengthens the lungs and eases tension in the upper back and the neck and shoulder region.

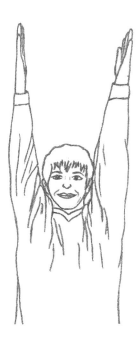

5.10 Clapping your hands above your head

Sit at the front of your chair. As you inhale, raise both arms out sideways and up to shoulder height. Then, as you exhale, raise your arms even higher, so as to clap your hands above your head. As you inhale, lower your arms back to shoulder height. As you exhale, clap your hands again above your head. Do this exercise five to seven times. Then bend over forwards, let your arms dangle and relax in this position for a few seconds. Slowly sit up again and feel the effect.

Effect
This exercise strengthens the heart.

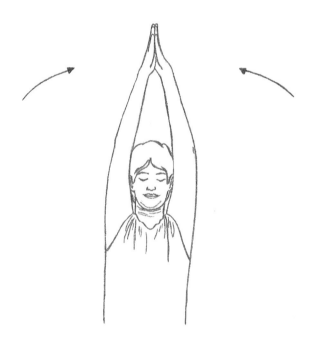

■ 5.11 Stretching the arms and letting them go

Sit at the front of your chair, with your knees and feet shoulder-width apart, and your feet directly underneath your knees. Raise your right arm in front of you and stretch it vertically upwards. On the next inhalation, stretch upwards with your arm. Briefly hold the stretch, and your breath. As you exhale, lower your right arm into your lap or down by your side. Do this three times with the right arm, three times with the left arm and three times with both arms. Feel the effect.

Effect

This exercise eases tension in the arms and stretches the muscles and tendons in the arms.

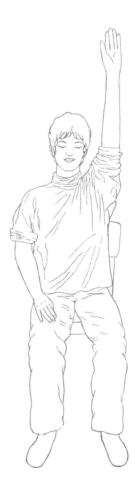

■ *5.12 Pushing the walls apart*

■ Take your arms out to the sides and up to shoulder height. Your hands are angled upwards, with the fingertips pointing upwards and the palms outwards.

■ Imagine that there are two walls to your right and left, and that the palms of your hands are touching them.

■ On the next inhalation, stretch outwards, hard, with your hands. Imagine that you are pushing the two walls apart.

■ As you exhale, let go.

■ Repeat this exercise three times. The third time you can stay in the stretch for a few breathing cycles.

■ Then, as you exhale, lower your arms, bend forwards and loosen up your arms if you need to. Sit up and feel the effect.

Effect

This exercise stretches the tendons and muscles of the arms and eases tension in the shoulders.

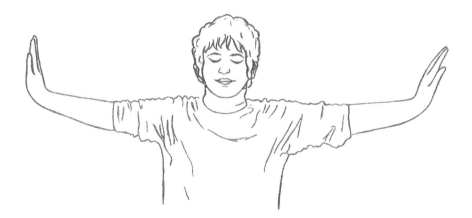

■ 5.13 Pushing weights

Sit at the front of your chair. Imagine that you have two heavy weights, one resting in your right hand and the other under your left hand. As you inhale, push the imaginary weights as hard as you can away from one another. As you exhale, let go, and lower the raised arm back down by your side.

Repeat twice more and then do it the other way round – left arm up, right arm down – three more times.

Effect

This exercise stretches the tendons and muscles of the arms and eases tension in the neck and shoulder region.

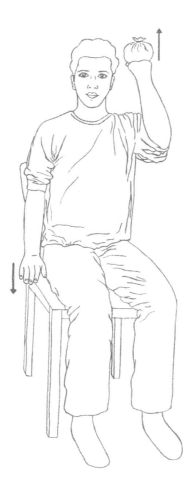

6

EXERCISES FOR THE BACK

In India the spine is called *Brahma Danda*, 'God's walking stick'. Our wellbeing stands and falls with its mobility. Someone who has constant back pain loses their *joie de vivre* – but if the spine is mobile and supple, then we feel young and full of élan. The main problem for our back is standing erect. If we were still running or crawling on four legs like animals, we wouldn't have backache.

The spine has many different tasks: it keeps us upright, absorbs impacts and burdens through the discs and, with the help of muscles, keeps the head balanced on the topmost vertebra. It keeps us upright, and any movement alters its balance. At the same time, inside the spinal canal, it protects sensitive nerve fibres that must be free of pressure. So it's worth doing something to keep our backs in good health.

Here too, the more the muscles carry, the less wear there is on the bones.

What does the back need in order to stay healthy? Movement.

It needs to bend forwards and backwards, and to bend and twist to right and left – and all this completely without stress, in peace, with deep breaths, so that the tissues have sufficient oxygen at all times. Each muscle must have time to transfer body weight to the next one. The back dislikes jolting, rapid movements as much as it dislikes long spells of sitting. Even just gentle swaying to and fro allows the back muscles to play, and provides them with fresh blood and oxygen.

Feel into your back. How does it feel? Does it stay upright by itself, or do you have trouble keeping it like that? Can you feel the muscles that hold up the spine, or do you rather feel that the bones are holding the muscles together?

Does the right side feel the same as the left? Or do you have a 'soft side'?

First, feel into the neck vertebrae…then those of the chest (or thorax)…the lumbar vertebrae…and finally the sacrum. Are they strong and in harmony, or do you have the feeling that somewhere there are blockages?

Take time to feel your back.

The benefits of back exercises are:

■ strengthening and relaxing the musculature of the back

■ stimulation of cleansing/clearing

■ freeing blockages in the nervous system

■ stronger circulation in the abdominal space and all the internal organs

■ increased flexibility of the spine.

Exercises for the back contribute to inner as well as outer uprightness.

■ 6.1 Dance pose (Natarajasana)

■ Sit on the front of your chair. Put your right foot a little way out in front, and your left foot a little way back.

■ Now, with your left hand, hold onto the back of the chair.

■ As you inhale, stretch your right arm vertically upwards and look up at your right hand. Stay in this stretch for three to ten breaths (depending on your ability).

■ As you exhale, slowly lower your right arm, take your left hand away from the back of the chair, bring your feet together and briefly let your arms dangle as you bend over forwards.

■ Stand up straight, briefly feel the effect and repeat the exercise on the other side.

Effect

This exercise strengthens the muscles of the back and arms, eases tension in the neck, shoulder and back areas and lengthens the spine.

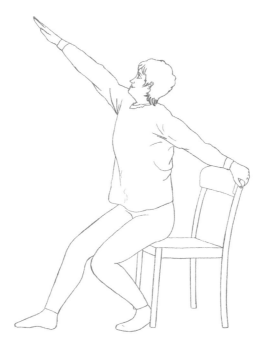

■ *6.2 Twisting forward bend*

Variation 1

- Sit on the front of your chair, with your knees shoulder-width apart.

- Lay your left forearm across your thighs, and shift most of your weight onto your left elbow.

- As you inhale, slowly raise your right arm out to the side and vertically upwards; look up at your right hand and let your breath flow.

- After three to nine breathing cycles, lower your right arm slowly as you exhale, release and lower your left arm as well, lean over forwards and let both arms dangle.

- Sit up straight again and feel the effect before doing the exercise with the other side.

Variation

Make a fist with the hand that is stretched upwards and then spread out the fingers. Do these alternative movements a few times.

Effect

This exercise eases tension in the back, shoulder and neck areas. In addition, 'pumping' (alternately making fists and spreading out the fingers) stimulates lymph flow in the upper body. The exercise broadens the chest and stimulates breathing.

Variation 2

- ▣ Link your hands at the back of your head. As you inhale, reach backwards with your elbows.

- ▣ As you breathe out, let your right elbow drop towards your right thigh (only as far as your body allows).

- ▣ As you inhale, sit up straight again and reach backwards with your elbows.

- ▣ As you exhale, let your left elbow drop towards your left thigh.

- ▣ Repeat twice more on each side. The last time you can stay in this position for three to five breaths.

Effect

This exercise eases tension in the back, shoulder and neck areas, broadens the chest and stimulates breathing.

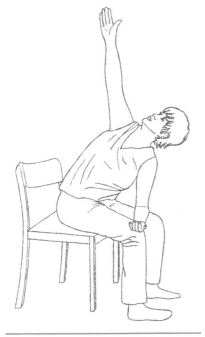

Variation 1

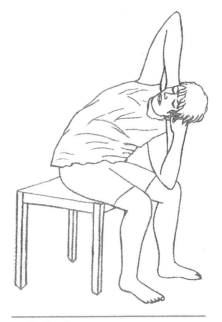

Variation 2

■ 6.3 Half spinal twist (Matsyendra Asana)

Be careful: If you have hip joint replacements, you should not cross your legs, as this can have a negative effect. Just keep your legs parallel with each other. You will find nevertheless that this exercise is very effective.

■ Slide slightly forward on your chair so that you are sitting freely with your back upright.

■ Cross your right leg over the left one, and place your left hand on the outside of your right knee.

■ Lay the back of your right hand horizontally across your lower back.

■ Keeping your upper body straight, twist to the right as you exhale, as far as your body allows. Let your breath flow.

■ To begin with, three to six breaths is long enough to remain in the twist position. Later, when you have more flexibility, you can stay longer in the twist position.

■ As you inhale, turn slowly back to the centre. As you exhale, move your right hand away from your back, and lower your right leg.

■ Briefly lean forward and let go of everything before doing the twist to the opposite side. Cross your left leg over the right one, place your right hand on your left knee and your left hand on your lower back and, as you exhale, twist to the left.

Effect

The vertical twist prevents stiffening and wear and tear of the spine. The sitting twist is one of the few movements that make the back mobile in the erect position. This in turn has a positive effect on the central nervous system, as the sensory and motor impulses that emanate from it can then flow unimpeded. The entire nervous system is kept fresh and lively. The abdominal organs are massaged and receive increased blood supply by means of alternate twisting of the body. Constipation is prevented or eliminated.

Variation

Instead of placing the back of your hand across your lower back, stretch your arm out to the side at shoulder level. In this way the shoulder and outstretched arm receive increased blood supply. Tension in the neck and shoulder region is gradually removed.

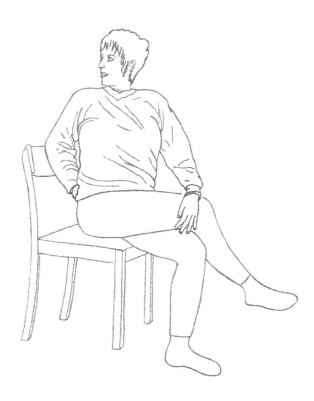

■ 6.4 Tiger breathing

■ Sit on the front of your chair and push your hands forwards onto your knees.

■ This movement sequence begins in the pelvis. As you inhale, tilt your pelvis forwards, then bend backwards, dropping your head back onto your neck.

■ As you exhale, tilt your pelvis backwards and arch your back in the manner of a cat. As you do so, direct your gaze towards your navel.

■ Do these movements slowly and with awareness, several times, in coordination with your breathing – about four to eight times.

■ Then let your arms dangle, sink forwards with your upper body and let go of everything.

■ Sit up slowly and feel consciously into your back.

Effect

This exercise keeps the spine supple, has a preventative and soothing effect on back pain and increases the power of concentration.

***

Be careful: If you have back trouble, don't go too far in hollowing your back. (You risk a prolapsed (slipped) disc!)

***

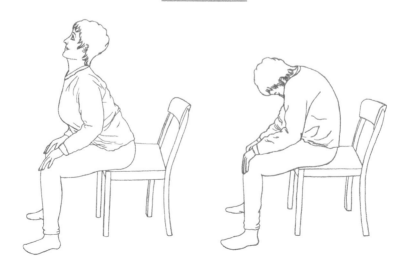

■ 6.5 *Back and arm extension*

Variation 1

■ Sit on the front of your chair. Your back is erect but relaxed. Link your hands behind your back.

■ As you inhale, pull your arms downwards, so that your shoulders are stretched back and your chest widens. Let your head drop very lightly back towards your neck.

■ As you exhale, loosen up. Your head and upper body are upright once more. Repeat this exercise twice more. Briefly notice how it feels before doing Variation 2.

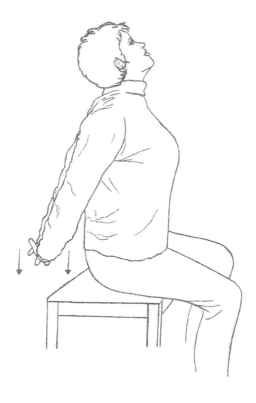

Variation 2

Bring your palms together behind your back and link your hands. Your upper body remains erect and straight. As you inhale, slowly and carefully stretch your linked hands upwards. Go only as far as the pain threshold. Hold the stretch, and your breath, very briefly. As you exhale, slowly lower your arms. Repeat the exercise twice more.

Effect

Both variations ease tension in the regions of the shoulders, neck and upper back, broaden the chest, stretch the shoulder muscles and stimulate the glands. They generate self-confidence.

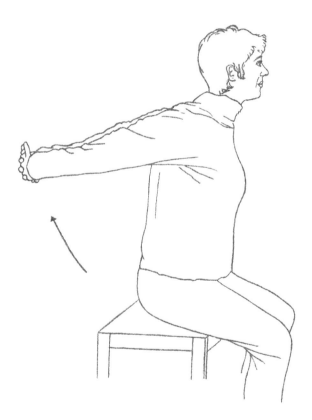

■ 6.6 *Spinal twist with arms bent*

■ Sit on the front of your chair. Link your hands behind your head and as you inhale, stretch your elbows a little backwards (only up to the pain threshold).

■ As you exhale, and keeping your upper body straight, twist to the right and look towards your right elbow.

■ As you inhale, turn back to the centre.

■ As you exhale, twist to the left; look towards your left elbow. Twist slowly, keeping to the rhythm of your own breathing, altogether three times to each side.

■ Then, on an inhalation, turn back to the centre; on the exhalation lower your arms, lean forward and let go of everything.

■ Sit up and feel into your shoulders, neck and upper back.

Variation

In the final twists you can linger for a few moments on either side and let your breathing flow.

Effect

This exercise eases tension in the upper back, neck and shoulder area, keeps the spine supple, strengthens upper chest breathing and has a positive effect on memory.

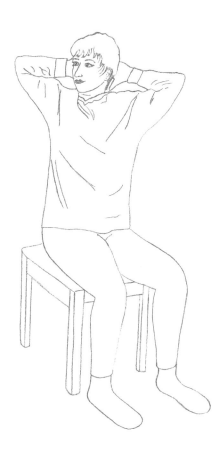

■ 6.7 *Spinal twist with outstretched arms*

■ Sit on the front of your chair. Cross your right leg over the left. Take your arms out to the sides and up to shoulder height.

■ As you inhale, turn your head to the right and look at your right hand.

■ As you exhale, turn your upper body to the right; your right arm is now (ideally) pointing backwards, and your left outstretched arm is pointing forwards.

■ Go as far into the twist as your body allows, without any forcing at all. Stay in the twist for three to six breathing cycles, continuing to look at your right hand.

■ As you inhale, turn your upper body and head slowly back to the centre.

■ As you exhale, lower your arms to your sides and uncross your right leg.

■ Now bend forwards and let your arms dangle.

■ Sit up, and after a short pause do the exercise for the other side of your body: the left leg over the right, arms out to the sides to shoulder level.

■ As you inhale, turn your head to the left and look at your left hand.

■ As you exhale, twist your upper body to the left.

■ Stay in the twist – depending on ability – for three to six breathing cycles. Enjoy noticing how it feels afterwards.

Effect

As for Exercise 6.6.

Be careful: If you have artificial hips, don't cross your legs!

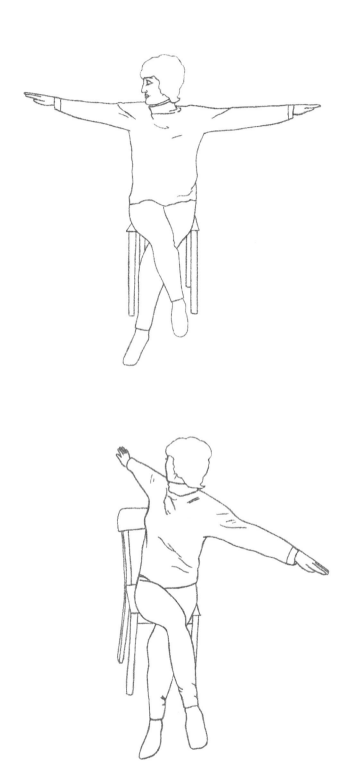

■ 6.8 Lateral extension

- ■ Sit on the front of your chair. Link your hands behind your head and stretch your elbows gently backwards.

- ■ On the next exhalation bend your upper body sideways to the left.

- ■ As you inhale, sit up; back to the centre.

- ■ Now as you exhale, bend your upper body to the right.

- ■ As you inhale, back to the centre.

- ■ Do the exercise three times to each side. Then, as you exhale, free your hands and bend forwards.

- ■ Let your arms dangle, and feel the effect.

Effect

This exercise strengthens the muscles of the back and shoulder blades, and the lateral muscles of the trunk. Lymph flow is stimulated.

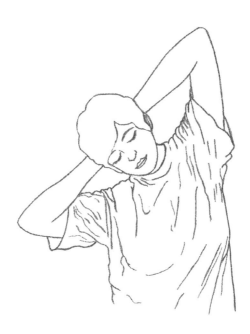

■ *6.9 Back flexion with leg extension*

- ■ For this exercise lean against the back of your chair. Place your hands by your sides, next to your thighs.

- ■ As you inhale, stretch your right leg out in front.

- ■ As you exhale, lean forwards with your upper body, as far as your body allows.

- ■ On the following inhalation raise your upper body; as you exhale, take your right leg back down.

- ■ Repeat the exercise twice more with your right leg and three times with the left.

- ■ Then place your hands on your thighs and feel consciously into your abdominal and pelvic area.

Effect

The exercise extends the back muscles and the muscles along the backs of the legs, strengthens the abdominal muscles and gathers lots of energy in the abdominal and pelvic regions.

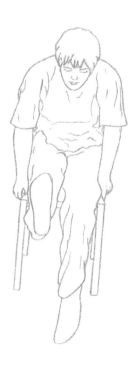

7

EXERCISES FOR
THE SHOULDERS,
THROAT AND NECK

The shoulders, throat and neck form the 'cross' of the human skeleton. They carry not only the head but every kind of load – our heavy shopping, as well as our cares. As a result this area in particular is often very tense. (Stubbornness may also have something to do with it.) So let's make the effort to turn our heads more freely, thus widening our horizons.

Building muscle is also important here. If the arm muscles are able to take the weight, then our wrist, elbow and shoulder joints don't get worn out so quickly. The same is true for the throat muscles: if they support the head and are well built up, the back of the neck doesn't need to be tense.

Sit upright and feel into your throat, neck and shoulders. Can energy flow freely, or does it feel dull and heavy? Is your spine straight?

Round your shoulders and feel how crooked your back is in this position.

Now let your shoulders drop back and lift your breastbone. Can you feel how your whole body straightens up, and your mind has a much more cheerful view of the world?

Observe your posture for the course of a day. Do you droop, or walk upright? What happens to your mood when you straighten up?

Benefits of the exercises for the neck and shoulder area:

■ Tension is released.

■ Circulation and the removal of waste products are improved.

■ Joints become better lubricated and more supple.

■ The thorax widens and allows more breathing space.

■ The muscles of the throat and chest grow stronger.

■ There is more room for peace of mind and mental 'space'.

7.1 Propeller

- Sit on the front of your chair. Your back should be straight and your shoulders loose.

- Turn your right palm up, and the left one down.

- Curl your fingers and then bring your hands together in such a way that the fingers of each hand can hook onto the fingers of the other.

- Inhale, and slowly raise your right elbow as far as your body allows (only as far as the pain threshold).

- Exhale and turn your arms in the opposite direction, like a propeller: now your left elbow will be pointing up, and the right one down.

- Raise each elbow three times, keeping your upper body straight. Only your arms and shoulders should move.

- Then link your hands and, as you inhale, stretch upwards with your arms, palms directed towards the ceiling; feel the stretch through your upper back, shoulders and arms.

- Either stay in the stretch for several breathing cycles or, on the next exhalation, relax your arms and lower them into your lap.

Effect

This exercise eases tension in the shoulders, neck and upper back.

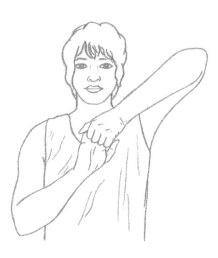

■ 7.2 Dropping the shoulders

Sit on the front of your chair, with a straight back. Let your arms hang by your sides. As you inhale, gently pull both shoulders up; as you exhale, gently let them drop, breathing out hard, or with a sigh, as you do so. Imagine that as you breathe out you are shedding all weight from your shoulders. Do this exercise three times.

You could follow through with the next two exercises.

Effect

This exercise eases tension in the neck and shoulders.

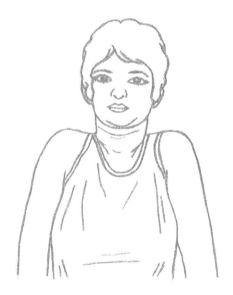

7.3 Circling with the shoulders

Variation 1

Place your right hand on your right shoulder, and your left hand on your left shoulder. Make big circles with your elbows, backwards and forwards, three or four times. Do these circular movements quite deliberately. Breathe normally as you do so.

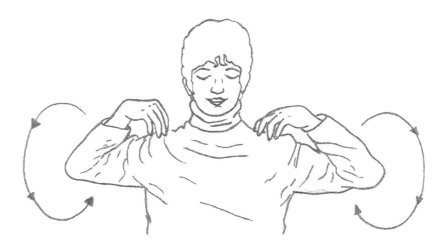

Variation 2

Continue with your arms hanging by your sides and now circle only with your right shoulder, about three times backwards and three times forwards. Then do the same with your left shoulder. Then circle with both shoulders, three times backwards and three times forwards. As you do the circling, try to be consciously in your shoulders.

Effect

This exercise eases tension in the neck and shoulder area and loosens the shoulder girdle.

■ 7.4 *Massaging the shoulders*

For this exercise you can either sit up straight on the front of your chair, or lean back comfortably.

Place your left hand on your right shoulder. Massage your right shoulder and the neck and throat area. Then make a fist with your left hand and tap gently with it all over your shoulder. Then lower your left hand into your lap. Now massage your left shoulder with your right hand. Tap with your fist all over your left shoulder.

Effect

This exercise eases tension in the neck and shoulder area.

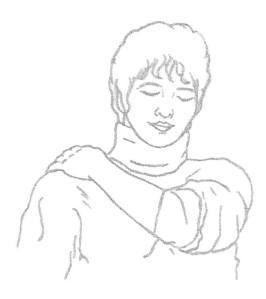

■ *7.5 Shoulder stretches*

■ Sit on the front of your chair with your back straight. Place your right hand on your right shoulder, and your left hand on your left shoulder.

■ As you exhale, stretch your elbows forwards so that, ideally, your elbows touch.

■ As you inhale, stretch your elbows back as far as your body allows.

■ Repeat three more times. Then lower your hands into your lap and briefly feel the effect.

■ Now place your hands on your shoulders again.

■ As you inhale, stretch your elbows upwards, and as you exhale, downwards – as far as you can, but only up to the pain threshold.

■ Repeat three more times.

Effect
This exercise eases tension in the neck and shoulder area.

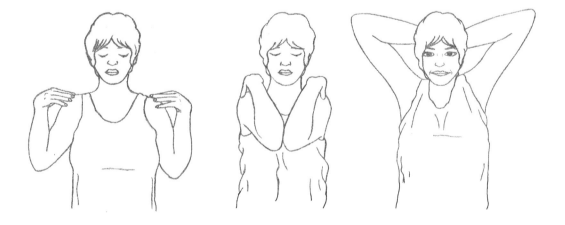

■ 7.6 *Head leaning to one side*

Let your head drop gently 'in slow motion' towards your right shoulder, and then just as slowly towards your left shoulder. Repeat twice or three times more.

Then look slowly over your right shoulder, and slowly over your left shoulder. Repeat another two or three times. As you do this, let your breathing flow quietly.

Take your head back to the centre and feel the effect.

Effect

This exercise stretches the muscles in the sides of the neck and eases tension in the front and back of the neck.

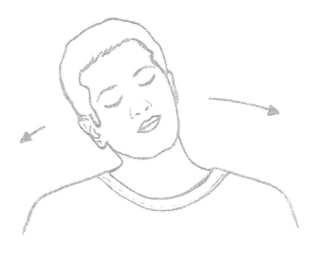

Be careful: Never do this exercise too quickly, or you may strain the muscles and vertebrae of the neck.

■ 7.7 Turning the head slowly (Brahma Mudra)

Variation 1

■ For this exercise you can sit back comfortably on your chair. Close your eyes.

■ As you inhale, turn your head very slowly towards your right shoulder, and as you exhale, turn your head very slowly towards your left shoulder.

■ Do this exercise three times. Then turn your head back to the centre.

■ Let your head drop gently towards the back of your neck (your lips can be slightly open); as you exhale, let your head drop gently forwards. Do this also three times.

■ Then turn your head back to the centre and feel consciously into the front and back of your neck.

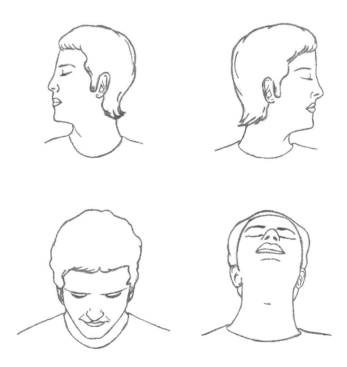

Variation 2

As you inhale, turn your head slowly towards your right shoulder, and as you exhale, back to the centre. As you inhale, turn your head slowly to the left – towards your left shoulder – and as you exhale, to the centre. Then, as you inhale, let your head drop towards the back of your neck, and as you exhale, to the centre. As you inhale, let your head drop forwards, and as you exhale, to the centre. Repeat twice more.

Effect

This exercise eases tension in the front and back of the neck and supports the functioning of the thyroid and parathyroid glands.

7.8 Shoulder rotation

Sit on the front of your chair, with space behind your back. Stretch out your arms at your sides and raise them to shoulder height. Your palms are turned upwards and your thumbs are extended away from the fingers. Breathe in. As you exhale, rotate your palms downwards, then back behind you, and upwards, as far as you can. As you inhale, rotate your hands back to the starting position. Repeat this rotation three to five times. Slowly lower your arms onto your lap.

For a more difficult variation, keep your hands in the fully rotated position for a few breathing cycles.

Effect

This exercise loosens the muscles around the shoulder joints, and keeps the latter supple. It eases tension in the neck and shoulder area.

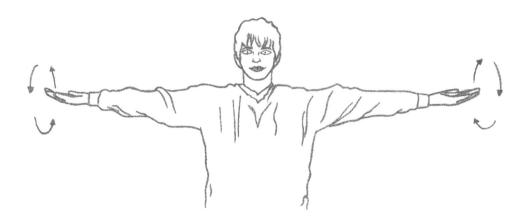

8

STANDING EXERCISES (SOME WITH A CHAIR, SOME WITHOUT)

Here, for the sake of variety, I introduce a few exercises that you can do standing – in some cases holding onto the chair to help you stay in balance.

In the course of daily activity it's very important to keep changing position. Doing nothing but sit all day is very harmful for the spine. It's better to have a change, at least once an hour, from sitting to standing, walking or lying. If you are obliged to sit for a long time, you should at least change your sitting position every so often, to stop your muscles from becoming rigid.

Rock a little to and fro, or from left to right. Bend over forwards, lean back against the backrest of your chair... Human beings need variety and movement. Give your muscles a chance to play.

In standing, the body feels different from the way it feels in sitting. Just feel this new position: I'm standing...

Your legs should be hip-width apart in order to give your body stable balance. Your shoulders are rolled slightly backwards. To avoid a hollow back, bend your knees ever so slightly, so that you can push your sacrum slightly forwards. This posture ensures that you are standing with the help of your leg muscles, and not with knees braced, just on the bones.

Now sway a little to the right and the left and feel how your back muscles come into play. Now the right side is bearing weight, and now the left. Find your preferred rhythm and decide for yourself when you have played for long enough.

Benefits of standing exercises

■ The intercostal muscles are stretched.

■ Ischial pain is prevented.

■ Lung capacity is increased and breathing improves.

■ Lymph flow is stimulated by muscle activity, detoxifying the body.

■ Physical and spiritual balance, and the integration of the two brain hemispheres, are strengthened.

■ Blood supply to the entire head region, especially the brain (concentration, memory) and eyes, is enhanced.

■ Tension in the pelvic area is eased.

■ 8.1 Half (or crescent) moon

■ Stand behind your chair. Your feet are shoulder-width apart, and you are standing up straight. Hold onto the back of the chair with your left hand.

■ As you inhale, slowly raise your outstretched right arm up over your head.

■ As you exhale, lean with your upper body gently over to the left, up to the pain threshold. (Your arm will make a slight curve above your head.)

■ On the next inhalation slowly stand up straight again and lengthen upwards.

■ As you exhale, lean over to the left again.

■ Repeat the exercise for a third time. On the last inhalation, keep your upper body erect, and as you exhale, slowly lower your right arm.

■ Now hold onto the back of the chair with your right hand. As you inhale, slowly raise your left arm.

■ As you exhale, lean over to the right.

■ Repeat the exercise twice on this side too. Then slowly lower your left arm.

■ After a brief pause to feel the effect, raise both arms out to the sides as you inhale, until they are vertical above your head.

■ As you exhale, lean over to the right.

■ As you inhale, back to the centre.

■ As you exhale, bend to the left, and so on.

■ Lean over three times on each side.

■ On the last inhalation stand up straight and, as you exhale, slowly lower your arms down to your sides. Feel consciously into your sides.

Effect

This exercise stretches the lateral muscles and prevents ischial pain, as the ischial nerve is stretched. Lower lung capacity is increased, that is, abdominal breathing is improved.

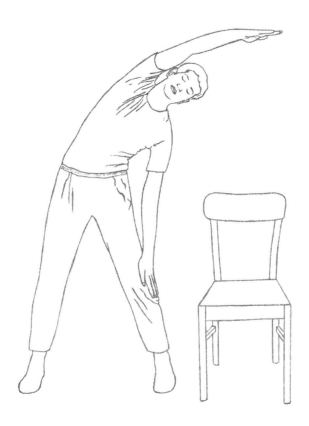

■ 8.2 The crane

For the rest of the exercises in this chapter we boldly dispense with the chair.

Stand with your feet shoulder-width apart and parallel with each other. Place one hand palm up inside the other. As you inhale, slowly raise your arms out to the sides and up, go up on tiptoe and let the backs of your hands briefly touch above your head. As you exhale, gently lower your arms down by your sides, and come smoothly back down onto the soles of your feet. Repeat this three to five times. As you exhale, slowly lower your arms back down by your sides.

Effect

This exercise has a harmonizing effect, opens out the ribcage, stimulates circulation and strengthens breathing.

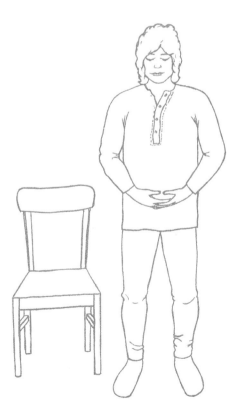

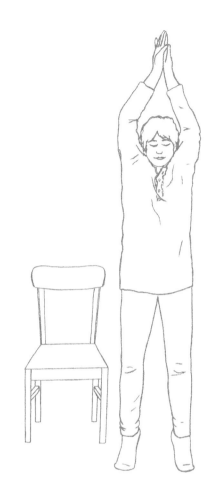

◼ 8.3 Walking with a spring in your step

Stand up straight with your legs slightly apart. Alternately lift your right and left heel, leaving the ball of the foot in contact with the floor. Your knees should be directed forwards, and your back straight. Imagine yourself light and loose, going on your way through the world with a light spring in your step and with upright posture, loose shoulders, your face relaxed and perhaps slightly smiling.

Effect

This exercise helps to maintain an upright posture (important for older people), and keeps the feet and toes supple.

■ 8.4 Circling the knees

Set your feet a little way apart. Take care that they are parallel with one another. Place your hands on your knees, or slightly above them, and bend them slightly. Now make circles with your knees. Do this circling movement slowly and deliberately. After circling for a bit in one direction, circle slowly the other way, five to ten times in each direction. Then stand up slowly. Loosen up in your legs.

Feel consciously into your knees.

Effect

This exercise eases tension in the knee joints and keeps them supple.

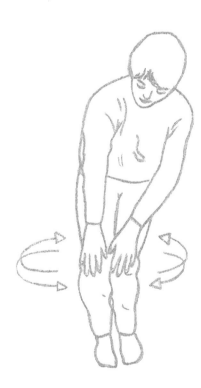

■ *8.5 Circling the hips*

Set your feet a little more than shoulder-width apart. Place your hands on your sides at about waist height and circle your pelvis, first about five times in one direction and then about five times in the other.

Then lower your arms and feel into your pelvis and lower back.

Effect

This exercise eases tension in the pelvic region.

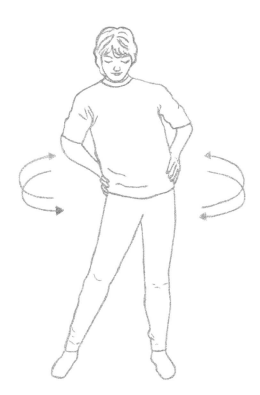

■ 8.6 Circling the upper body

Raise your arms sideways and up over your head until the palms of your hands meet. Now, with your arms and upper body together (and keeping your upper arms close to your ears), make circles, small ones to begin with, in one direction. As you circle, your upstretched arms and upper body should form a single line. Make your circles gradually larger, but only so big as to let you keep your balance. Then circle the other way. Make your circles gradually smaller again, until you are back at your starting point.

Then lower your arms by your sides and enjoy feeling the effect.

If necessary, this exercise can also easily be done sitting on the front of your chair.

Effect

This exercise eases tension in the back, neck and shoulder areas and stimulates the flow of lymph in the upper part of the body.

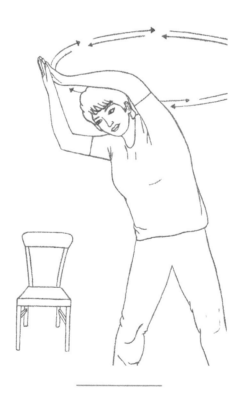

Be careful: If you have lower back problems you should only do this exercise if circling doesn't cause you any pain.

8.7 Variation on standing twist (Dola Dolati, 'pendulum')

■ Stand upright, with your legs and feet as wide apart as possible. Stretch out your arms at shoulder height.

■ As you inhale, turn your head to the right and look at your right hand.

■ As you exhale, turn the whole of the upper part of your body to the right. Your feet can also twist a little to the right, but keep the soles firmly on the floor.

■ As you inhale, turn your head and upper body back to the centre.

■ As you exhale, turn your head and upper body to the left (and look at your left hand).

■ On the following inhalation, turn back to the centre.

■ As you exhale, turn to the right. Take care that your pelvis is turning too.

Do this exercise several times to each side, keeping your arms at shoulder height and stretching them out as far as possible. If your arms get tired, lower them, and to the rhythm of your own breathing, turn a few more times from one side to the other. As you do so, blink hard. When you want to finish the exercise, stay at the centre as you exhale, and let your arms drop back to your sides. Bring your feet back to about shoulder-width apart, and go on to the second part of the exercise.

■ Place the palms of your hands on the outside of your thighs.

■ Sway gently from one foot to the other, and blink gently.

■ After swaying from one side to the other for a while, remain at the centre, close your eyes and feel the effect.

Effect

The first part eases tension in the neck and shoulder area and the back, and keeps the spine supple; the second part calms the nerves and senses.

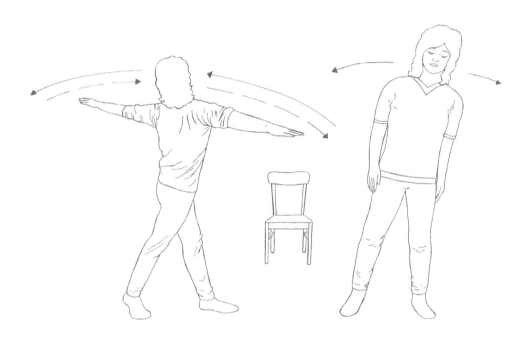

9

EXERCISES FOR BOTH SIDES OF THE BRAIN

The human brain consists of several parts. The oldest part is the 'reptilian brain' in the back of the head, directly above the first neck vertebra, which controls our breathing and survival. In the course of evolution new parts of the brain were continually added; and finally, just behind the forehead, the forebrain with its left and right hemispheres. Here is the part that makes us human, that makes it possible for us to reflect, remember and invent. Not in vain do we speak of the domed 'thinker's forehead'.

The left brain hemisphere is home to logical, mathematical thought, short-term memory and newly learned skills.

In the right brain hemisphere are the faculties of *gestalt* and creative thinking, long-term memory and skills learned in the distant past.

If, for example, I am learning to drive, I do it first with the left brain. After I have had some practice and don't have to think about what to do all the time, I control the car with my right brain, and there is space once more in the left brain for learning something new. It's the same with everything that people learn: swimming, riding a bicycle, languages...

These examples show why the cooperation of both sides of the brain is so important: the short-term memory would become overloaded and unable to take in anything more if it could not pass on its newly acquired information to the long-term memory. Conversely, I need to be able to retrieve old information in order to learn new rules, otherwise I become forgetful. Many people can't remember where they put a key a minute ago, but remember exactly where they used to put it 30 years ago. Here the link between short- and long-term memory has been disrupted.

It's not only for memory and learning that we need this collaboration between the two brain hemispheres, but also for harmonious movement. The left brain steers the movement of the right side of the body, and the right brain that of the left side.

Hence scientists have learned that cross-patterning exercises are especially good for the brain, because the two hemispheres are forced to work together. You move your left arm and right leg, for example, or your right foot and left hand.

If you would like to get your brain in training, take a good look at the following exercises and try them out. To begin with, the movements may seem very complicated because it's a long time since your body has done any cross-patterning exercises. But rest assured. It will get used to them. Here too, practice makes perfect.

■ 9.1 'Clang' exercise

Sit on the front of your chair. Stretch your arms straight out in front of you, with the palms of your hands turned upwards. Inhale deeply, and as you exhale, sing 'Clang', with the emphasis on the 'ng', and at the same time slowly open your arms out to the sides. Briefly lower your hands into your lap. Repeat once or twice more.

Effect

This exercise makes the sinuses vibrate and has a positive effect on mood.

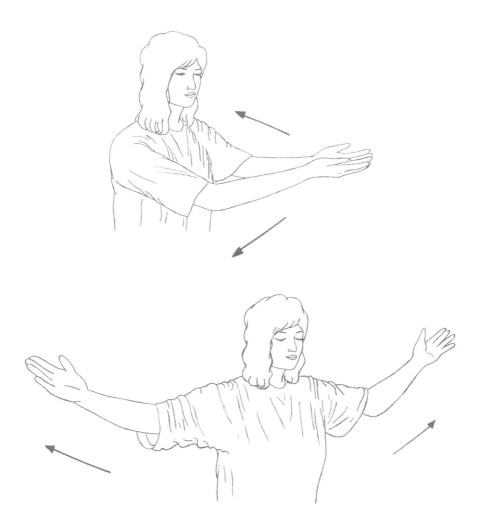

■ 9.2 'Gong' exercise

Stretch your arms straight out in front of you, with the palms of your hands turned upwards. Inhale deeply and, as you exhale, sing 'Gong' and make a big circle with your arms, from the top down. Repeat this exercise once or twice more.

Effect

This exercise makes the sinuses vibrate and has a positive effect on mood.

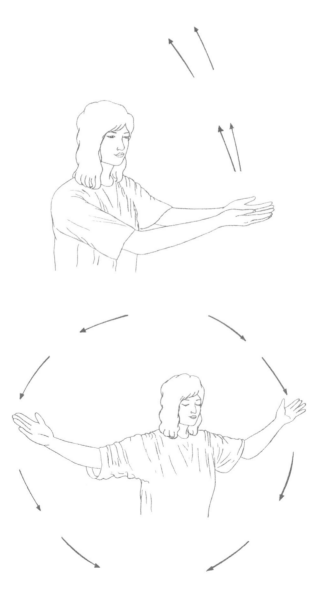

9.3 Raising opposite arm and leg

For this exercise you can sit with your back against the chair, or upright on the front of the chair.

As you inhale, stretch your left leg and right arm out in front of you. As you exhale, slowly lower your arm and leg. Do the same with your right leg and left arm.

Do this exercise about ten times each way.

Effect

This exercise coordinates the two halves of the brain and strengthens the arm and leg muscles.

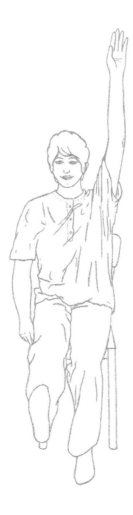

■ *9.4 Hand-to-knee cross-patterning exercise*

Variation 1

For this exercise sit on the edge of your chair. Raise your left knee a little and briefly tap your right hand on your left knee. Then raise your right knee and briefly tap your left hand on your right knee.

Repeat this 20 to 40 times.

You can also do the exercise more quickly.

Effect

This exercise coordinates the two halves of the brain and increases the power of concentration.

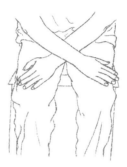

Variation

Put your left hand on your left knee and your right hand on your right knee. The knees are about shoulder-width apart. Then bring your knees together at the centre, at which point change hands, putting your left hand briefly on your right knee and your right hand briefly on your left knee. When you open your knees again, put your right hand back on your right knee and your left hand back on your left knee.

Repeat this 10 to 20 times, alternately crossing the right hand over the left, and the left hand over the right. If you are doing well, do it faster from time to time.

Effect

As above.

■ 9.5 *Balancing pose*

Place your feet about shoulder-width apart. Transfer your body weight to your right foot. Slowly raise your right arm and look at a fixed point on the ground. Slowly take your left foot off the ground. If this is too difficult, the big toe can stay in contact with the ground. Your left palm should be touching the outside of your left thigh. Try to stay in this balancing pose and let your breath flow quietly (about three to five breathing cycles). As you exhale, slowly lower your left foot and your right arm. Close your eyes and feel the effect before doing the exercise on the other side.

Effect

This exercise improves your sense of balance.

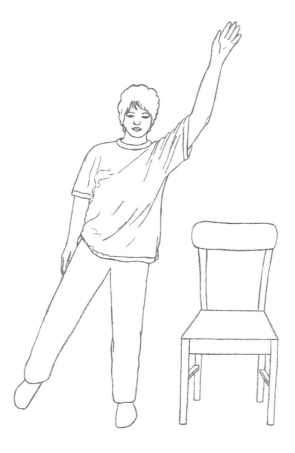

■ 9.6 *Horizontal figure of eight*

You can do this exercise sitting or standing.

Take your arms up over your head and swing them in a horizontal figure of eight; first a few times to the right, then to the left.

Effect

This exercise coordinates the two halves of the brain and eases tension in the neck and shoulder area.

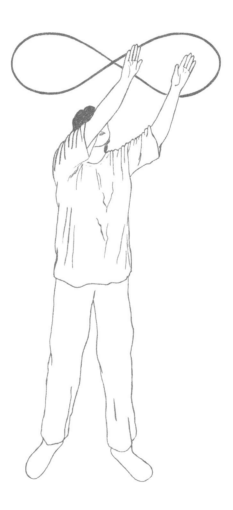

10

PELVIC FLOOR EXERCISE

Most people think about pelvic floor exercises only in connection with antenatal training, but the pelvic floor has an altogether different dimension. Not only does its tension keep the abdominal organs in place, preventing prolapse of the bladder and uterus, but it also has a key influence on the postural aspect of the spine. From yoga we know that toning the pelvic floor releases positive life forces, letting the sun shine in the soul.

But what exactly is it?

The pelvic floor consists of several layers of muscles that close up the base of the bony pelvis. On it rests the weight of the innards contained in the abdominal space. It has to be able to withstand this pressure. Therefore it is constructed from three layers of muscle that close the pelvis like a grille and have only three apertures: the orifices of the bowel (anus), urethra and vagina.

The outer layer of the pelvic floor is in the form of a horizontal figure of eight, in the front part of which are the urethra, clitoris and vagina, and in the back part the anus.

If the pelvic floor is weak, it can lead to organ prolapses and urinary incontinence, especially when you cough or sneeze. To prevent this, you can train your pelvic floor.

Sit up straight on your chair and feel into your pelvis. First notice your two sit bones in contact with the chair. Shift a little to left and right in order to feel them more distinctly.

Then shift to and fro, and once again feel where and how the base of your pelvis makes contact with the chair.

Imagine a figure eight on the floor of your pelvis.

Now take this eight by the centre and gently pull it up, as if you were picking a handkerchief up off the floor.

Once more: inhale and gently pull the pelvic floor up, and as you exhale, slowly(!) release it. You can also imagine a lift going slowly up, and just as slowly back down. A wonderful feeling. Once you have mastered this, try a more difficult method in which you hold the tension as you exhale, so that this muscle group can be conditioned even more. Hold the tension for one or two breaths and then, on an exhalation, let it go.

Are you still having difficulty finding the right muscles?

Then try it on the toilet. Try consciously to interrupt the flow of urine by means of muscle power, and then let it flow again. Can you close off the urethra completely?

You can do this pelvic floor exercise, tensing and letting go, frequently in the course of the day, as well as in a yoga session. Practise as you read, watch TV, stand in the checkout queue at the supermarket. Take advantage, whenever you are waiting anywhere, to strengthen your pelvic floor. Your back, your bladder and your psyche will thank you for it.

Advanced students can go further: tense your pelvic floor and hold the tension for three or four breathing cycles and then, on an exhalation, release.

Note that although the introduction and exercise in this chapter focus on the female anatomy, pelvic floor exercises can also be used effectively by men.

A few more tips

Pelvic floor problems affect women in particular, because their muscles and ligaments are softer than men's. Pregnancies put pressure on the pelvic floor, because the child is resting on it.

Avoid unnecessary strain. Don't carry any heavy objects.

When you are carrying something, hold it as close to your body as you can.

To stoop down, bend your knees slightly.

Never stand with your legs together. Your feet should always be hip-width apart.

Stand upright; don't hollow your back.

Strengthen your breathing (taking advantage of the effect that breathing has on the lower abdomen).

Sit up straight.

Here is another summary of the exercise.

10.1 Tensing the muscles of the pelvic floor

As you inhale, squeeze your buttocks together hard and pull your anus upwards. As you exhale, release. Do this at least ten times. The last time (with a bit of practice) you can try letting your breathing flow as you keep the pelvic floor muscles tensed for three or four breaths.

Effect

This exercise is especially suitable for women. It prevents prolapse of the bladder and uterus and has a positive effect on mood.

11

EXERCISES FOR THE EYES

If the blood supply to the eyes deteriorates, so does our vision – so good upper lung breathing (see the chapter on breathing exercises), and exercises that condition the blood vessels in the head region, are important.

The eyes have always played a large role for humans. At one time it was important to be able to spot dangers as early as possible, so as to be able to fight or flee. Nowadays the things we want to see are smaller; we want to be able to recognize letters, whether in a book in front of our nose or on a road sign 100 metres away. That is a big challenge. Most demanding for the eyes is focusing for hours at the same distance, as happens on long car journeys, or when we sit for hours in front of the TV or a computer. The eyes get tired.

The eye muscles need to be exercised, just like all the other muscles in the body. Otherwise they get flabby. Only when a muscle moves does it get fresh blood and fresh oxygen. Being still for too long means getting out of condition. Let's be aware that the eye also has muscles that require exercise.

Close your eyes and feel into them. Are they peaceful and relaxed, or are your eyelashes quivering a bit?

Take a few deep breaths. Then turn your 'inner gaze' to the centre of your forehead. Feel how this relaxes the eyes. All the crows' feet are smoothed away.

Open your eyes and look all the way to the right, then all the way to the left (six times).

Without moving your head, look down as far as you can, then up as far as you can (six times).

Now look at an object that is quite close to you; and then at one that is quite a long way away, preferably outside the window (six times).

Now move your eyes in circles, three times to the right and three times to the left.

Close your eyes again, and feel into them. How do your eyes feel now?

Here are the benefits of the following yoga exercises for the eyes:

- The optic nerve is strengthened.

- The eye muscles are exercised.

- The eyes relax.

- Lymph flow is stimulated in the head region.

- The power of concentration improves.

- The eyes become more mobile and receive better blood supply.

For the following exercises you can make yourself comfortable with your back against the backrest of your chair. You can do the exercises one after the other.

11.1 Energizing the eyes

Energize your hands by rubbing the palms vigorously together until they feel hot. Now put your hands over your closed eyes, slightly hollowing your hands. Can you feel the warmth and energy emanating from your hands? Keep your eyes closed, and repeat the process of rubbing your hands and putting them over your eyes twice more. Then, still with your eyes closed, lower your hands into your lap.

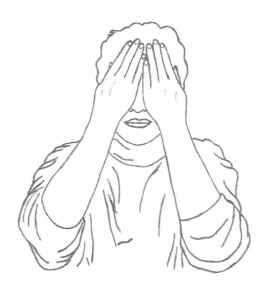

11.2 Head and face massage

■ Put your hands on your head and massage the scalp with your fingertips, as if washing your hair.

■ Then tap your fingertips very gently over your scalp.

■ Then lay the index and middle fingers of both hands on the bridge of your nose and stroke, with gentle pressure, over your eyebrows to the temples. Stroke higher and higher in the direction of the hairline, so that you stroke over the whole of your forehead.

■ Then rub in circles a few times over your temples.

■ Finally, with your index and middle fingers, rub gently in front of and behind your ears. Don't do this too fast.

■ Then massage the outer edges of your ears and, gently, the flaps of the ears.

■ Gently tug the earlobes, three times.

■ Then, with all of your fingers, massage your throat and the back of your neck. Stroke from the hairline downwards and to the sides.

■ Then lower your hands comfortably into your lap. After 10 to 20 seconds to feel the effect, you can open your eyes slowly.

Effect

This exercise strengthens the optic nerve, and relaxes the eyes and the muscles of the face and the back of the neck. It supports the functioning of the lymph nodes in the neck area. As this exercise has a very calming effect, it is a good one to do before relaxation.

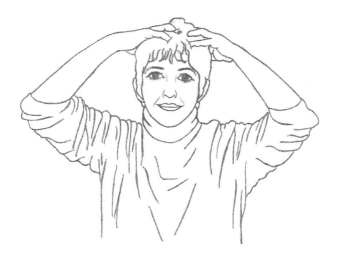

■ *11.3 Circling around a dot*

Raise your right arm, stretching it out in front of you, to eye level and extend your right index finger. In your mind's eye, point to a dot. Now circle your index finger slowly around the imaginary dot. Let your gaze follow your finger. Gradually make your circles larger. Then circle in the opposite direction. Make your circles smaller again, until you have mentally arrived back at the starting point.

After closing your eyes briefly, repeat the exercise with your left index finger.

Effect

This exercise increases the power of concentration, and is good for your eyes.

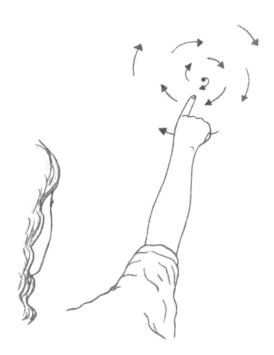

11.4 Watching a pendulum

Close your eyes and imagine a large, white wall. Against this white wall you can see a pendulum constantly swinging from right to left and back. Follow the movement of the pendulum with your eyes a few times, slowly, from one side to the other. Your head can swing very lightly along with it. Then let the pendulum movement come to a standstill. Keep your eyes closed and feel the effect.

Effect

This exercise relaxes the muscles of the eyes.

■ 11.5 Exercising the eyes

Rub your hands together until they are pleasantly warm. Now put your hands over your closed eyes, slightly hollowing the palms. Leave your hands over your eyes. With the eyelids closed, look slowly three times upwards to the right, and three times downwards to the left. Keep your eyes closed. Rub your hands together again and then look three time upwards to the left, and three times downwards to the right. Rub your hands one last time and move your eyes (behind closed lids) in circles, three times slowly to the right, and three times slowly to the left.

Lower your hands into your lap and enjoy feeling the effect.

Effect

This exercise strengthens the muscles of the eyes, keeps the eyes mobile and strengthens the optic nerve.

12

RELAXATION

Most people nowadays are plagued by stress. The body is tense and the mind is restless. At this level of stress the body can neither digest food properly nor recover. The immune system is weakened and the person is constantly tired, weak and breathless and lacking drive. The body and mind don't have time to sort themselves out internally, to separate good from bad and 'find space' for wellbeing.

In order to stop this process and re-activate the 'physician within', it's important to give yourself time to relax every day. A good time for this is the middle of the day, as the body's energy is lower at this time and it is very thankful for a rest.

You can use the relaxation techniques in this chapter either by yourself in the middle of the day, in the evening before you go to bed or as part of a yoga programme of your choice (see Chapter 13). Time for rest after yoga is particularly important, as during this time the effects of the exercises develop. Through the yoga exercises energy is guided back into the right channels, and it should have the chance to 'tick over' for a while before you return to your daily routine and all its challenges.

In relaxation 'the body enters the alpha state', according to those who do research into sleep. This means that in the course of everyday activity we are running on very high frequencies, but during relaxation we are within the bandwidth of calm. It's like a radio that has been retuned from rock music to a relaxing flute concerto. This alpha vibration not only takes care of relaxation but also sets back in motion the digestive processes, which require rest, gives the heart a rest and more oxygen and boosts the immune system. Often you come out of relaxation more refreshed than you are after a midday snooze.

Just as important as sinking gently into relaxation is returning from it peacefully. After relaxing for a little while, breathe deeply in and out a few times. Then stretch the way you do when getting out of bed: stretch and then dangle your arms, stretch and relax your legs. Move each finger individually, open and shut your eyes a few times and blink at the world once more, as friendly, alert and active as a squirrel.

Conscious relaxation

Sit comfortably on your chair, lean against the backrest but take care that your back is straight. Your hands are resting loosely in your lap. Focus on the waves of breathing in your abdomen. Consciously feel your abdomen slowly rising as you inhale, and slowly sinking as you exhale. Let yourself be carried on your breath, the way a great sea carries many little waves. With each exhalation let your thoughts grow calmer, let go of the external world and sink deeper and deeper into your own world. Go systematically through your body from your feet upwards, consciously relaxing the various areas of the body.

Afterwards we inhale deeply and exhale deeply. We extend and stretch, as we do on waking up, and as we exhale we let go fully once again, lean over forwards, let our arms dangle. We extend and stretch once or twice more, and let go.

As we inhale we straighten up slowly.

Relax your feet.	My feet are completely relaxed.
Relax your ankles.	My ankles are completely relaxed.
Relax your calves and knees.	My calves and knees are completely relaxed.
Relax your thighs.	My thighs are completely relaxed.
Relax your bottom.	My bottom is completely relaxed.
Relax your pelvic region.	My pelvic region is completely relaxed.
Relax your abdomen.	My abdomen is completely relaxed.
The abdomen is warm and soft.	My abdomen is warm and soft.

The chest is wide and free.	My chest is wide and free.
Relax your lower back and around your sacrum.	My lower back is completely relaxed.
In your thoughts, ascend your spine like a staircase and relax the vertebrae one at a time.	In my thoughts I am ascending my spine like a staircase, relaxing the vertebrae one at a time. My whole back is relaxed.
Both your shoulders relax, your upper arms, elbows and forearms, your hands.	My shoulders are relaxed. My upper arms, elbows and forearms, both my hands are relaxed, right into the tips of my fingers.
Relax each of your fingers, right into the fingertips.	
Relax your neck and throat area, the back of your head, your ears, your forehead, which is quite smooth, your eyes, which are gently closed.	My neck and throat are completely relaxed. The back of my head, my ears, my forehead, which is quite smooth, my eyes, which are gently closed.
Relax the many little muscles around your eyes.	
Relax your nose, cheeks and mouth.	My nose is relaxed, my cheeks, my mouth. My lips are warm and very soft. My tongue is resting loosely inside my mouth. My face is very peaceful and joyful.
Let go of all thinking, all wanting, all having to, and sink into the middle of your forehead. Think about nothing at all; just be.	I am letting go of all thinking, all wanting, all having to, and sinking into the middle of my forehead. I am thinking about nothing at all.

■ *Leading a yoga group*

This text should be spoken slowly. Leave a slight pause after each paragraph.

We are thinking about our feet, may they always carry us lovingly, our feet are completely relaxed.

We are thinking about our ankles, may they always be supple. Our ankles are completely relaxed.

Our calves are completely relaxed, our knees, our thighs.

Our bottom is completely relaxed. We feel our bottom in contact with the chair, and we feel the chair carrying us, and the earth carrying the chair. And so every time we exhale, we can let go a little more. We are being carried. Then we relax our entire pelvic area and our abdomen. Our abdomen is very warm and soft, very relaxed. We can feel the natural rise and fall of our abdomen as we breathe in and out.

Then we relax our chest. Our chest is very wide and very free. Our breath flows very easily into us, and very easily back out again.

We think about the internal organs in our chest and abdomen, and about them working in there. All our organs are relaxing.

Then we relax the whole of our lower back, and around our sacrum. In our thoughts we are climbing, like climbing a staircase, relaxing the vertebrae one at a time. We are also relaxing all the muscles in our back, relaxing our shoulders. We are letting everything that is heavy on our shoulders slide off. We are freeing ourselves from everything that makes our life difficult, simply giving it up. We are acknowledging that now we are responsible only for ourselves and not for anyone else. Then we relax our upper arms, elbows, forearms and hands, relaxing each and every finger, right into the tips of our fingers.

Then we relax our neck and throat, the back of our head, our ears, our forehead, which is very smooth. All the worry lines are being smoothed away.

Our eyes are completely relaxed, the eyelids, the eyeballs, and also the many little muscles around our eyes.

Our nose is relaxed, our cheeks, which are very loose, and our mouth. Our tongue is lying very loosely in our mouth, our lips are warm and soft.

We are letting go of all thinking, all wanting, all having to. We have only the feeling of being a light, floating feather that is being carried in a warm summer wind.

We are flowing with life, flowing with the light, letting ourselves be led, letting happen, thinking about nothing any more. Simply being…! [Short pause – one or two minutes.]

We breathe in and out deeply. We extend and stretch as if waking up, and as we exhale we let everything go once more, bend over forwards, letting our arms dangle. We extend and stretch once or twice more and let go. As we inhale, we straighten up slowly.

13

EXERCISE GUIDELINES

▪ *Planning a chair yoga session*

Before embarking on any exercises, you should first stretch and extend vigorously, as when you wake up. This livens you up, stretches the spine and inner organs and stimulates improved energy flow in the body.

If, after that, you do the breathing exercises as well, your thoughts can calm down and your body benefits from a supply of fresh oxygen right at the beginning of your yoga session.

The sequence of exercises that you can now do should always begin with the lower body and work upwards. This has a positive effect on circulation and the activity of the heart.

First, I will give you suggestions for 15 minutes' exercise. These programmes are ideal for beginners and might be appropriate, for example, for those of you who are office workers, and/or for getting started at home.

Later I will give you suggestions for sessions of 30, 45 and up to 60 minutes, depending on how intensively you would like to practise yoga. You can, of course, also put together your own programme, using your favourite exercises.

If you find that you enjoy doing the exercises but lack the self-discipline that's required to do them on your own at home, then look for a yoga teacher whose approach you enjoy. Yoga should never be serious, nor even be done under duress. The important thing is for the group to feel at ease with their teacher, and also to have fun practising.

Do each programme that I propose to you every day for at least a week, so that body and mind grow accustomed to the exercise sequence. It's better to keep repeating a familiar programme and fully enjoy the exercises than to be constantly reorientating yourself as you leaf through the book. In the first place, readjusting always means stress for body and mind. If you know the programme, the familiarity enables you to let go more quickly. It's similar with horses that have practised their dressage routine hundreds of times. They can do it almost without direction from the rider – and our yoga exercises should be just the same: flowing, as if of themselves, without effort, strain or stress.

Please don't forget the rest after each exercise. It's better to do a 10-minute programme in peace and quiet than a 30-minute one in a flurry.

And now I wish you much fun with yoga!

Fifteen-minute yoga programmes

Programme 1

■ Extending and stretching/breathing exercises

■ Loosening and spreading the toes (2.5)

■ Clenching the toes (2.6)

■ Bicycling (3.7)

■ Half spinal twist (6.3)

■ Dropping the shoulders (7.2)

■ Circling with the shoulders (7.3, Variation 1)

■ Relaxation

Programme 2

- Extending and stretching/breathing exercises
- Rocking on the soles of the feet (2.2)
- Pushing the knees sideways (3.1)
- Spreading out the fingers/making fists (4.8)
- Spinal twist with arms bent (6.6)
- Tensing the muscles of the pelvic floor (10.1)
- Making circles with the arms (5.1, Variation 1)
- Massaging the shoulders (7.4)
- Relaxation

Programme 3

- Extending and stretching/breathing exercises
- Waking up the feet (2.4)
- Stimulating lymph flow in the lower part of the body (3.8)
- Tiger breathing (6.4)
- Locking the fingers together (4.3)
- Pressing the palms of the hands together (4.4)
- Extending the elbows (5.2)
- Spinal twist with outstretched arms (6.7)
- Relaxation

Programme 4

- ■ Extending and stretching/breathing exercises
- ■ Stretching the feet (2.7)
- ■ Wind-releasing exercise (3.5)
- ■ Clapping under the legs (3.6)
- ■ 'PAH' exercise (5.8)
- ■ Dance pose (6.1)
- ■ Energizing the eyes (11.1)
- ■ Relaxation

■ *Thirty-minute yoga programmes*

Programme 1

- ■ Extending and stretching/breathing exercises
- ■ 'Clang' exercise (9.1)
- ■ 'Gong' exercise (9.2)
- ■ Rocking on the soles of the feet (2.2)
- ■ Rolling the feet (2.3)
- ■ Bicycling (3.7)
- ■ Opening the hands (4.9)
- ■ The bud (4.10)
- ■ Bending the wrists (4.12)
- ■ Relaxing the ribcage (5.4)

■ Tensing the muscles of the pelvic floor (10.1)

■ Mountain pose (5.9, Variation 1)

■ Spinal twist with arms bent (6.6)

■ Lateral extension (6.8)

■ Shoulder stretches (7.5)

■ Turning the head slowly (7.7)

■ Head and face massage (11.2)

■ Relaxation

Programme 2 (with standing exercises)

■ Extending and stretching/breathing exercises

[Stand up]

■ Walking with a spring in your step (8.3)

■ Circling the knees (8.4)

■ Circling the hips (8.5)

■ Variation on standing twist (8.7)

■ Balancing pose (9.5)

[Sit down]

■ Tensing the muscles of the pelvic floor (10.1)

■ Spreading out the fingers/making fists (4.8)

■ Crossing your arms (5.5)

■ Propeller (7.1)

■ Relaxation

Programme 3

- ▪ Extending and stretching/breathing exercises
- ▪ Rolling the feet (2.3)
- ▪ Loosening and spreading the toes (2.5)
- ▪ Pushing the knees sideways (3.1)
- ▪ Massaging the legs (3.2)
- ▪ Bending the legs (3.3)
- ▪ Bicycling (3.7)
- ▪ Locking the fingers together (4.3)
- ▪ Pressing the palms of the hands together (4.4)
- ▪ Moving all the fingers separately (4.5)
- ▪ Harmonizing exercise (5.7)
- ▪ Twisting forward bend (6.2)
- ▪ Massaging the shoulders (7.4)
- ▪ Shoulder rotation (7.8)
- ▪ Energizing the eyes (11.1)
- ▪ Exercising the eyes (11.5)

Programme 4 (with standing exercises)

- ▪ Extending and stretching/breathing exercises

[Stand up]

- ▪ The crane (8.2)
- ▪ Half moon (8.1)

■ Balancing pose (9.5)

■ Horizontal figure of eight (9.6)

[Sit down]

■ Moving all the fingers separately (4.5)

■ Making circles with the fingers (4.6)

■ Half spinal twist (6.3)

■ Clapping your hands above your head (5.10)

■ Pushing weights (5.13)

■ Turning the head slowly (7.7)

■ Massaging the shoulders (7.4)

■ Relaxation

■ *Forty-five-minute programmes*

Programme 1

■ Extending and stretching/breathing exercises

■ Waking up the feet (2.4)

■ Rolling the feet (2.3)

■ Massaging the legs (3.2)

■ Loosening and spreading the toes (2.5)

■ Clenching the toes (2.6)

■ Pushing the knees sideways (3.1)

■ Wind-releasing exercise (3.5)

▪ Bicycling (3.7)

▪ Hand-to-knee cross-patterning exercise (9.4)

▪ Stretching the hands (4.13)

▪ Locking the fingers together (4.3)

▪ Pressing the palms of the hands together (4.4)

▪ Making circles with the arms (5.1, Variation 2)

▪ Bending the wrists (4.12)

▪ Extending the elbows (5.2)

▪ Circling around a dot (11.3)

▪ Relaxing the ribcage (5.4)

▪ Half spinal twist (6.3)

▪ Lateral extension (6.8)

▪ Propeller (7.1)

▪ Dropping the shoulders (7.2)

▪ Circling with the shoulders (7.3, Variation 1)

▪ Head leaning to one side (7.6)

▪ Energizing the eyes (11.1)

▪ Exercising the eyes (11.5)

▪ Relaxation

Programme 2

▪ Extending and stretching/breathing exercises

▪ Raising the heels (2.1)

- Loosening and spreading the toes (2.5)

- Clenching the toes (2.6)

- Making circles with the heels (3.4)

- Raising opposite arm and leg (9.3)

- Relaxing the ribcage (5.4)

- 'PAH' exercise (5.8)

- Pushing the walls apart (5.12)

- The bud (4.10)

- Moving all the fingers separately (4.5)

- Exercise for the wrists (4.11)

- Boat pose (3.9, Variations 1 and 2)

- Making circles with the arms (5.1, Variation 2)

- Tiger breathing (6.4)

- Half spinal twist (6.3)

- Circling with the shoulders (7.3, Variation 2)

- Shoulder stretches (7.5)

- Spinal twist with arms bent (6.6)

- Mountain pose (5.9, Variation 2)

- Energizing the eyes (11.1)

- Head and face massage (11.2)

- Relaxation

Programme 3 (with standing exercises)

■ Extending and stretching/breathing exercises

■ Rocking on the soles of the feet (2.2)

■ Waking up the feet (2.4)

■ Stretching the feet (2.7)

■ Bending the legs (3.3)

■ Boat pose (3.9, Variation 1 and 2)

■ Stretching the arms and letting them go (5.11)

■ Clapping your hands above your head (5.10)

■ Opening the hands (4.9)

■ Interlacing the fingers (4.1)

■ Shoulder rotation (7.8)

■ Tiger breathing (6.4)

■ Dance pose (6.1)

[Stand up]

■ The crane (8.2)

■ Circling the knees (8.4)

■ Variation on standing twist (8.7)

■ Balancing pose (9.5)

[Sit down]

■ Massaging the shoulders (7.4)

■ Turning the head slowly (7.7)

■ Relaxation

Programme 4 (with standing exercises)

▪ Extending and stretching/breathing exercises

[Stand up]

▪ Variation on standing twist (8.7)

▪ Circling the knees (8.4)

▪ Circling the hips (8.5)

▪ Horizontal figure of eight (9.6)

▪ Walking with a spring in your step (8.3)

[Sit down]

▪ Rocking on the soles of the feet (2.2)

▪ Waking up the feet (2.4)

▪ Bicycling (3.7)

▪ Making circles with the fingers (4.6)

▪ Spreading out the fingers/making fists (4.8)

▪ Stretching the hands (4.13)

▪ Interlacing the fingers (4.1)

▪ Making circles with the arms (5.1, Variation 1)

▪ Relaxing the ribcage (5.4)

▪ Spinal twist with arms bent (6.6)

▪ Lateral extension (6.8)

▪ Back flexion with leg extension (6.9)

▪ Turning the head slowly (7.7)

▪ Energizing the eyes (11.1)

■ Head and face massage (11.2)

■ Watching a pendulum (11.4)

■ Relaxation

Sixty-minute programme

■ Extending and stretching/breathing exercises

■ Own choice of exercises for the feet (2.1–2.7)

■ Massaging the legs (3.2)

■ Bending the legs (3.3)

■ Bicycling (3.7)

■ Harmonizing exercise (5.7)

■ Locking the fingers together (4.3)

■ Pressing the fingertips together (4.2)

■ Moving all the fingers separately (4.5)

■ Opening the hands (4.9)

■ Stretching the hands (4.13)

■ Making circles with the arms (5.1, Variation 1)

■ Crossing your arms (5.5)

■ Twisting forward bend (6.2, Variation 2)

■ Half spinal twist (6.3)

■ Stretching the arms and letting them go (5.11)

■ Tensing the muscles of the pelvic floor (10.1)

■ Tiger breathing (6.4)

■ Propeller (7.1)

■ Widening the chest (5.3)

■ Lateral extension (6.8)

■ Mountain pose (5.9, Variation 2)

■ Dance pose (6.1)

[Stand up]

■ Walking with a spring in your step (8.3)

■ The crane (8.2)

■ Half moon (8.1)

■ Variation on standing twist (8.7)

■ Horizontal figure of eight (9.6)

[Sit down]

■ Turning the head slowly (7.7)

■ Relaxation

■ Energizing the eyes (11.1)

■ Head and face massage (11.2)

■ Watching a pendulum (11.4)

■ Clapping under the legs (3.6)

■ Massaging the shoulders (7.4)

■ Circling the shoulders (7.3, Variation 2)

■ Spinal twist with arms bent (6.6)

MORE ABOUT YOGA

What is the secret of yoga? Why are millions of people still involved with such an old doctrine today?

As already mentioned in the introduction, the history of yoga goes back over 5000 years. The word 'yoga' comes from the old Sanskrit word *yui*, meaning 'yoke'. On the one hand, a yoke requires discipline, and so it imposes restrictions, ruling out many paths; on the other hand, it makes possible the union of two different powers. If a cart is to be pulled, then two horses with different personalities have to keep pace with one another. I am referring here to body and spirit. Only when they are evenly matched, vibrating in harmony, can a human being attain perfection.

Yoga is not a religion, even though the yoga path is closely linked with belief in reincarnation. Yoga has rules for the body and rules for the mind. These rules serve the sole purpose of developing people to their full potential, thus sparing them hard lessons in the next life. The goal is perfection, becoming one with God, once lessons have been learned, all bad habits 'worked off'. So we can understand yoga as the path of personal development, of working on oneself, on spirit and body, long before all the Greeks' philosophy.

To begin with, yoga was an oral tradition. There existed only a few old papyri in the shrines of the learned. The oldest depiction of a yoga pose was found on a stone seal that was made about 2500 BC. Yoga is also mentioned in the oldest mythological poems of India, the *Upanishads*, where it says: 'When the five senses and the mind are quiet, then the highest path of wisdom begins.' Concentration of the senses and quiet in the mind play a very big role in yoga.

In the third century BC the *Bhagavad Gita* was composed. It is part of the great Indian epic, the *Mahabharata*, and describes the problems that the warrior Arjuna met on his yoga path. His spiritual director and teacher is the god Shiva himself. Shiva shows Arjuna the three main yoga paths: *Jnana Yoga*

(Path of Wisdom, for those who love to study), *Karma Yoga* (Path of Action, of selfless service and assistance) and *Bhakti Yoga* (Path of Love and Worshipping God, akin to the monastic life). All these paths, however different, lead to the same goal: becoming one with God. The *Bhagavad Gita* makes clear that yoga is a practical path. Arjuna is an entirely 'normal' person, who goes on his way and asks questions like any other. He has human problems, bad habits and doubts. One of the main tenets of yoga is: You don't have to have faith; try it out and discover how it works on your own body.

▌ THE 'EIGHT-FOLD PATH'

The classical yoga tradition begins with the Yoga Sutras of Patanjali, at the time of Christ's birth. Patanjali describes the so-called 'eight-fold path'.

The physical exercises (*Asanas*) are the third level of this eight-fold path. Before embarking on it, one should concern oneself with Levels 1 and 2, the *Yamas* and *Niyamas*, ten ethical and moral rules that resemble the Christian Ten Commandments. They ensure that yoga is done with purity of heart and soul.

▉ 1. Yamas *(general restrictions)*

Non-violence (Ahimsa)

Ahimsa means that we should do no harm to any other creatures, whether in thought, words or deed. It requires us to practise tolerance towards other living beings; to accept the opinions of our fellow humans, even if we cannot share them; to develop understanding for the otherness of each and every person. It includes reconciliation, reduction of tension and the furthering of personal and interpersonal understanding. In conflict situations we should neither dwell on feelings of hate and dislike, nor want to force solutions by artificial means.

Truth (Satya)

Satya means not only speaking the truth, but living it as well. Deep truth is only known through deep inner unmasking of the things within us that are destructive and arrogant. It includes the realization that every other person is holding a mirror up to us – especially those who make our life difficult. We can develop the courage that we need in order to face up to these sides of ourselves again and again, without losing faith in positive transformation.

It is no use to anyone if we persist in a vicious circle of punishment, punishing ourselves in the way that perhaps our parents, teachers or others in authority used to do. We should not judge ourselves too harshly. When we become aware of our faults and weaknesses, we should pardon ourselves and learn from them. Sometimes we learn only through mistakes or suffering. Someone who is able to forgive him- or herself is able to forgive others more easily as well.

Not stealing (Asteya)

You should never take from anyone what doesn't belong to you. This includes showing others the recognition they deserve, for example for a well-done piece of work. This satisfies the deep human need for recognition and leads to increased effort and increased pleasure.

Control of sensuality (Bramacharya)

This means avoiding sexual egoism. We should not wish to possess the people and things we claim to love. *Bramacharya* is a call to practise acceptance of our fellow human beings – especially those close to us – just as they are – with the goal of one day being able to love them as well, just the way they are.

There are people who live *Bramacharya* in celibacy. These people have set themselves the goal of becoming pure in mind and deed. They consciously renounce sexual relations in order to devote themselves entirely to the pure love of God.

Non-possessiveness, generosity (Aparigraha)

This means curbing the desire for what is 'mine'. It means transcending egotistical grasping after worldly things, to reach an attitude of trusting that at an appropriate time we will receive what we really need. It presupposes that we will recognize so-called 'heavenly gifts', for they come not only in their own time but also – as the Chinese oracle, the *I-Ching*, says – in their own clothing. There is deep meaning in reaching a mental state of peace, so that we can open ourselves to the beneficent powers of the universe. We can be thankful every day for all that is positive and beautiful in our lives.

If we love, or think that we love, we often tend to turn the object of our love into a possession, whether it be our partner, our family, our work, our country…perhaps even our love of God.

The desire to possess blocks off the other person's positive response. This leads to tension and frustration between people, to the point of dislike and hatred.

■ 2. Niyamas *(observances)*

The second level is the *Niyamas*, or ethical rules. Here there are five precepts to aspire to on the spiritual level.

Purity *(Saucha)*

We should not only keep our body clear of harmful pleasures, but also be pure in mind. Observe your thoughts consistently for several hours. How many positive and how many less positive thoughts did you have? How often do you feel rage, revenge, fear of not getting the things that you are convinced you are entitled to? Check for yourself:

How many doubts attacked you, how many self-accusations? How much did you worry about things over which you have no influence?

All our thoughts affect the way we feel at every moment.

'Purity of thought' can also mean consciously practising positive thinking, repeating affirmations softly or aloud, learning to trust, praying, practising meditation. We should learn to be the master/mistress of our thoughts, and not their slave.

In a broader sense, *Saucha* also entails withdrawal from contacts that are harmful to us. If people around us do not want to change, we should keep our distance, without giving up on these people in our minds because of 'the way they are'.

We should also be critical in our choice of which books and magazines to read, and which films to watch. The things we do in our leisure time have a powerful impact on our thinking. It is up to each one of us whether we fortify ourselves with positive forces or deliver ourselves up to negative ones that will keep impoverishing us psychologically.

Contentment (Santosha)

We should regularly allow ourselves time for rest, so as not to be carried away by the hustle and bustle of our daily lives. If, increasingly, we find our own centre, then we will recognize that peace exists in the midst of confusion, light in the midst of darkness, life in the midst of death, truth in the midst of falsehood.

People who discover this for themselves develop the power and courage to free themselves from many old fears, worries and doubts. One's mind can become quiet, one's disposition cheerful and happy. The aura of such a person has a beneficial effect on others.

Developing inner fire: ardour, or spiritually motivated discipline (Tapas)

Tapas means the ability to exist 'in the here and now', having the discipline to be punctual, to develop regularity and reliability. *Tapas* also comprises willingness to review and, if need be, correct one's own point of view and feelings in interpersonal relations, in order to bring about greater understanding.

Further, *Tapas* also means developing the discipline to maintain our physical and mental health – for example, by regularly doing yoga, or taking exercise outdoors. In addition, we should avoid food and pleasures which we know to be harmful.

Self-knowledge through inner vision (Swadhyaya)

Swadhyaya is the search for knowledge of the self and willingness to let go of illusions, even though this can be painful. We all harbour many illusions in order to make our life more bearable – but these often get in the way between us and our fellow human beings. We easily project our wishes and hopes onto others (especially those close to us). This leads to many conflicts in interpersonal relations. If we are willing to become more conscious of our projections, many of our relationships can become less tense. It also comprises the insight that enables us to make positive changes in the things over which we have some influence, and to let go of those over which we have none.

Devotion to God (Atman Pranidad)

Atman Pranidad means discerning one's own inner consciousness, internal reality, true nature. It can also be interpreted as devotion to God and the ability to take seriously the divine spark within oneself.

■ 3. Asana *(pose, posture)*

We stand up erect and straight, or sit erect and straight. Stability increases in us. That is already an *Asana*, the third level. The *Asana* begins when effort stops and bliss occurs.

■ 4. Pranayama *(extension of the breath / energy)*

We feel the breath, follow it in our mind, guide it through our hands or with our mind to specific regions of our lungs or body (see Chapter 1 for breathing exercises) and control it.

■ 5. Pratyahara *(withdrawal of the senses)*

This is more difficult. I have to practise for a long time before I reach the point of really feeling only my breath in an *Asana*, without at the same time feeling, hearing, seeing, tasting, smelling my environment as well. So noisy neighbours can be a challenge. Can I turn my hearing away from them and only listen into myself?

■ 6. Dharana *(concentration / composure)*

Once we have succeeded in withdrawing our senses from the world and becoming oblivious to our environment, then comes composure of our inner powers. Now we let go of our own thoughts too; draw our mind inwards, to the centre. The objective is not to think anything any more, simply to be.

■ 7. Dyana *(meditation / higher awareness)*

There is an expanding inner consciousness of the 'I am'. All feelings and thoughts lie far behind us. Deep quietness reigns in the mind.

■ 8. Samadhi *(being-at-one, ecstasy)*

The feeling of 'I am' becomes a feeling of 'I am infinity'. I am you and he/she and animal and plant and stone and God. I am everything. I am part of the whole, like a raindrop that has merged first with the river, and now with the ocean. Ultimate happiness begins; ecstasy, bliss.

But at this level one does not rest. It is only a momentary state of enlightenment that demands of us that we work on ourselves over and over again, and means going back to Levels 1 and 2, the *Yamas* and *Niyamas*. Yet it is not really going back, for now we can see these laws in a new perspective. So it is more of an upward spiral movement, as in a mandala, a path on which we keep re-encountering old acquaintances and experiencing them in different ways. In this way we activate old powers that were formerly engaged in repressing banished material. These powers are now available for our continuing development; from the sediment comes energy for growth, just as, in a compost heap, new life arises out of that which is over.

What did one of my teachers once say? 'The task of the teacher is to keep rinsing out the vase and stirring the water in it, until there is no more sediment.' It can take a long time to work on ourselves until there is only clear water flowing within us.

Over the centuries different systems of yoga developed. The one that is most widespread in the West is Hatha yoga. The concept comes from the Sanskrit. *Ha* means 'sun' – positively charged, golden energy – and *Tha* means 'moon' – negatively charged, silver energy. It is a matter of keeping these two polar forces in balance. Hatha yoga works to achieve this balance with exercises, breathing and meditation. With poorly trained teachers this can turn into a form of gymnastics, which at best will benefit the body but has no effect on the mind/spirit or the energy system.

Genuine yoga exercises always work on all three levels: body, mind and spirit. They strengthen the vital force and give the psyche a positive boost as well. It is a question not only of building up muscle but of stimulating the whole metabolism; suppleness and stability; concentrating thought, energy and vitality; balancing relaxation and exertion. At the end of a good yoga session one feels well rested, in spite of having done a lot.

■ *DIET*

The sages who developed the yoga poses (*Asanas*) by means of observing animals also discovered that an animal's diet is a key factor in determining its character and its health. Cats, which are predators and eat meat, are restless, constantly on the move. Herbivores have a more relaxed lifestyle, chewing all day long and fighting only if attacked, and they have a significantly higher life expectancy than carnivores. So it became clear that a vegetarian diet is conducive to a peaceful, contemplative mind and good emotional balance. Animals thrive best when they are feeding on the plants that grow in their environment, according to season. They eat the plants unprocessed, raw; so the yogis did the same.

But the human race has developed. Our soils are overcultivated, we live protected from nature in houses and cities. We move around less than our ancestors and do scarcely any physical work, and the climate is colder than in India.

Raw food suits only a very few people. We need the warming energy of fire in order to endure the autumn, winter and early spring. Keeping animals is also an important part of human history, which ensured survival in winter. A mainly meat-free diet that takes animal suffering into account is certainly something to aim for, but not a fundamental condition for following the yoga path.

The same is true for alcohol, coffee, medications, nicotine and other drugs. Nothing is forbidden. But someone who is in sympathy with their own body and with animals will, for the most part, renounce recreational poisons, and will not voluntarily inflict harm on themselves or others. The more we feel what is good in ourselves and our diet, the greater becomes our desire for what generates this sense of wellbeing. Let the body decide what it needs. Offer it fresh fruit and vegetables every day, whether raw or cooked, and you will feel it doing you good. Offer it the goodness of wholegrain cereals – and from time to time give it some naughty little treat as well! The important thing is to listen to your body, so as to hear the gentle inner voice, and to feel what gives you energy and what doesn't. Diet is a very personal matter. Everyone needs to find out for themselves what does them good.

■ *The right diet – not just for reasons of health*

Foodstuffs in the natural state have a fundamentally more positive impact on your emotional and physical health than preserved ones.

Freshly harvested foods contain not only the most vitamins and minerals, but also *Prana*, the elemental vital force that we receive not only from our food, but through respiration, from the air! The older a foodstuff is, the less it contains of vitamins, minerals and *Prana*. Preserved foods contain the least. Therefore it's recommended to consume vegetables, for example, when they are as fresh as possible. If braised or steamed, they should still be crunchy, to preserve as much vitamin content as possible. If you can digest it easily, eat raw food as often as you can – ideally every day. But do so only in the morning, at lunchtime or in the afternoon. In the evening raw vegetables – although they are light – can be indigestible. Here too, listen to your body. Raw food will suit you to a greater or lesser extent depending on what 'type' of person you are.

■ *Why organic foods are preferable to those produced by conventional agricultural methods*

Essentially, it's better to buy food from an organic supplier or health store, as conventionally produced foods, despite 'looking better', are full of pesticides.

Apart from that, by purchasing food that has been chemically treated you are supporting further contamination of the Earth, since monoculture and intensive animal farming continue to develop as a result of ever-increasing agricultural production. Ecological balance has been increasingly destroyed. Plants in their 'cultivated forms' can only survive thanks to substances that protect them (pesticides) and destroy insects (insecticides), fungal diseases (fungicides) and wild plants (herbicides).

Organic agriculture, on the other hand, not only produces unsprayed food, but makes an important contribution to environmental conservation. Its main concern is not to exploit the soil, but to take care of it. Sensitive management of the soil preserves the mini- and micro-organisms that are responsible for producing humus. Mixed cropping restricts the spread of harmful organisms and increases the resistance of plants as well – so the spraying of herbicides, insecticides and pesticides can be abandoned. Organic manures provide balanced food for the soil and support the vitality of soil organisms. Finally, the sequence of crop rotation preserves the soil from the demands of monoculture, and giving up chemical fertilizers protects our water. Mineral fertilizer is rejected because it causes disharmony in the balance of soil nutrients and disturbs or kills off soil organisms.

Natural biotopes create space for helpful creatures and protect the food supply of birds and bees. Aromatic herbs and flowers grown in the immediate proximity of vulnerable crops can serve as a biological defence, providing natural repellents.

Monoculture or conventional agriculture, on the other hand, cause pollution of the water table. Mothers are already advised not to use mains water for preparing formula or baby food.

With increased awareness you, as a consumer, can foster the organic farming methods of the future, since protecting our own health encompasses the need to keep our environment healthy.

▨ *Why whole foods are more nutritious and health-giving than foods made with refined flour*

Whole foods offer protection from diseases in which diet is a factor, such as heart and circulatory conditions, digestive disorders, tooth and gum problems and cancer, to name but a few. Whole foods increase vitality, improve your looks, increase performance and cleanse congested tissue.

Cereal products provide energy, protein, carbohydrates, iron, calcium and thiamine (Vitamin B1). The wholegrain and its outer layers contain proteins, minerals and vitamins, which are lost in the milling process. The nutritional value of white flour is therefore significantly less than that of brown flour.

As technology advanced in the course of the nineteenth century, flour was milled not just as it was needed, but also to be stored. In order for it to 'keep', the wheat germ and the outer layers of the grain were removed, as these are what causes the rancid and musty taste of flour that remains in storage for long periods.

The loss of essential nutrients in the milling process is very high:

Essential nutrients	Loss as a result of milling
Vitamin B1	86%
Vitamin B2	69%
Vitamin B6	50%
Niacin	86%
Vitamin E	100%
Iron	84%
Copper	75%
Magnesium	52%
Calcium	77%
Manganese	72%

Furthermore, wholegrains, along with vegetables, legumes, fruit and nuts, provide the roughage that is so important for digestion. Many of the diseases of modern civilization, such as chronic constipation, heart disease, bowel cancer, diseases of the metabolism and of the blood vessels, are closely linked with lack of dietary fibre.

Fibre swells up, fills the stomach and intestines and produces a lasting sense of being full. It keeps you slim, as it uses up energy for metabolism. It binds toxins, produces smooth stools and creates the conditions for healthy intestinal flora – for many diseases have their origin in the intestines. Fibre also has the property of binding cholesterol in the intestines, preventing cholesterol build-up in the body and damage to blood vessels. A well-regulated digestion cleanses connective tissue and firms up the face.

The nutrition-reformer Kollath calls nutrition lacking in essential nutrients 'mesotrophy – semi-nutrition'. It leads to semi-health, for being healthy means being pain-free. In our competitive society very many people suffer from listlessness, lack of drive, sleep disturbance, depression, nervous disorders, digestive complaints, headaches… For people who are overweight there is the risk of additional illnesses such as, for example, raised cholesterol levels, joint and respiratory problems, diabetes, gallstones, cirrhosis of the liver. One in three people dies of heart and circulatory disease. Bad nutrition causes plaques on the walls of blood vessels; as a result the heart does not receive sufficient oxygen, heart function deteriorates and blood pressure rises.

Why we should think again about eating meat

If you do yoga regularly and take an interest in healthy nutrition, that does not mean that you have to go vegetarian. However, there are a few aspects to meat consumption that are worth considering.

Meat is a source of high-quality protein, but over and above a certain regularly consumed amount, this produces an excess of protein within the human body. Toxic by-products of protein – in particular uric acid, which can cause gout and rheumatism – lead to disturbed metabolism at high levels of meat consumption. Besides, meat contains all the waste and metabolic residue of the slaughtered animal, which are always toxic and act like poisons in the human body. With high consumption of meat, fish and eggs, putrescent processes take place in the human alimentary canal; these can lead to constipation.

■ 'Rich people's meat is poor people's hunger'

If we, the populations of industrial nations, were to go back to a more plant-based diet, we could succeed in the fight against world hunger. Nonsense? Have you ever stopped to think how much grass a cow eats before it is fully grown and slaughtered? If that ground were cultivated for grain, vegetables, fruit, etc., it would feed far more people than the few kilograms of meat provided by a dead cow.

Consider that we keep three times more animals for meat in the world than there are people living in it. These animals all have to be fed, so that their flesh can ultimately be eaten by humans. At the same time, two-thirds of humankind are starving.

Absurd, too, is the fact that third-world countries are obliged to export valuable sources of protein for us to use as feed for our pigs.

Veterinary medicines are not given only to sick animals nowadays; they are mainly administered to healthy animals. In order to produce more meat with less food, hormones are administered – this saves up to a third of expenditure on feed. Tranquillizing and neuroleptic medication is given for stress relief during transport. Many medications are broken down in the animal's body, others are stored in the liver and kidneys and remain as residue in animal-derived foods.

Anyone who nevertheless likes eating meat would do well to buy meat and sausage from an organic butcher, to guarantee at least that the animals have been reared and fed in a more or less appropriate manner. Picture to yourself how cruel intensive farming, transport and artificially accelerated growth are for animals. The same is true for eggs and dairy products: intensive poultry farming is just as wrong as feeding animal-based meal to calves.

The first commandment of yoga philosophy is *Ahimsa* – non-violence! Be aware that every creature also has the right to live.

■ *Sprouting seeds – green shoots from grain*

Seed sprouts are essential for good nutrition. The shoots are germinated grains – a nutritious fresh food, and guaranteed organic produce. Grain and seeds are store-cupboards full of nutritive energy. They deliver nutrients in concentrated form, because the substances latent in the grain are activated during germination. They provide us with high-quality proteins, essential fatty acids, minerals, trace elements and vitamins, all in a unique organic balance, just as our body needs. All kinds of cereals are suitable for sprouting (at the whole food shop ask explicitly for cereal that is suitable for sprouting): green soya beans, mustard seeds, cress and radish seeds.

With a handful of shoots and sprouts we can cater for our daily essential requirement of vital substances in a natural way, just as efficiently as by using meat, milk and eggs. Vitamin supplements become redundant.

Why sugar is harmful

According to the World Health Organization,[1] the average person in Europe consumes 107.3g of sugar per day, including 96.8g of refined sugar and 1.3g of honey. Strict nutritional experts consider 60g to be a just about acceptable amount.

It is true that sugar beet, from which sugar is produced, contains Vitamin B1, which is essential for metabolism of carbohydrates – but it is destroyed by the refining process. This makes white household sugar a so-called 'empty' carbohydrate containing neither vitamins nor minerals, but only calories.

The Japanese physician Dr Katose has discovered that sugar 'steals' calcium. Compared to other children, those who eat too many sweets present more frequently with physical damage in the form of reduced bone density, bone deformities and damage to the spine.

Sugar can cause addictions. This can lead to various disorders, some minor, others more serious, including irritability, hypersensitivity and severe mood swings. It is helpful to observe yourself whenever your desire for something sweet increases. Do you enjoy your square of chocolate, or do you stuff yourself full of it in order to avoid having certain feelings?

If you have a sweet tooth, try replacing chocolate with dried fruit, or a piece of fresh fruit according to season – for example, strawberries, cherries, apples… Mangos, papayas and pineapples are also on offer, but in these cases we need to take account of 'air miles'.

---

1   World Health Organization (2003) *GEMS/Food Regional Diets: Regional per Capita Consumption of Raw and Semi-processed Agricultural Commodities.* Available at www.who.int/foodsafety/chem/gems_regional_diet.pdf, accessed on 19 July 2011.

A good alternative to sugar is honey, as it is a natural sweetener. Honey contains substances that split carbohydrates, thereby assisting the metabolism. It also inhibits the growth of harmful bacteria and stimulates circulation through the coronary blood vessels. Honey is one of the 'cleanest' of foods and is easily digestible. It is a fast source of energy, as its sugar content enters the bloodstream in a matter of minutes without any digestive process.

Another alternative to sugar is maple syrup, which comes from wild maple trees. It contains vitamins and minerals. Birch syrup and fructose can also be recommended as sweeteners.

Brown sugar is not a genuine alternative to white sugar, as its mineral and vitamin content is insignificant.

Be aware that it takes time to make changes. Don't be too strict with yourself, but don't lose sight of your goals. Dietary habits that are harmful to health can't be broken in a flash. Observe what suits your digestion. Each person has a preference for particular foods, and there is no reason to eat something you don't like just because it's good for your body.

■ *Nuts*

Nuts are among the most valuable sources of concentrated protein and fat. They deliver energy and contain large amounts of Vitamin B.

If you regularly eat raw, unsalted nuts, meat is an unnecessary food, even if you are doing heavy physical work. This is especially true if you give up sugar and refined flour products and eat plenty of fruit and vegetables. In the fresh, raw and unsalted state, almonds are the most alkaline of all nuts. They are valuable as food for the bones and for strengthening tooth enamel.

Nuts that have been cooked, roasted or in any way exposed to very high heat levels have a negative effect on our organism as a result of changes that these conditions bring about in fat: then there is a harmful effect on the liver and gallbladder, such that the functioning of these organs could sooner or later be impaired.

Nuts are best eaten fresh, and between meals. It is beneficial to combine them with carrot juice. On no account should nuts be eaten at the end of a heavy meal, on account of their high percentage of protein and fat.

Water

Although water, strictly speaking, is not a food, it is essential for life, as all metabolic processes can only take place with water. Lack of fluid causes headaches, nausea, impaired performance, exhaustion, unpleasant body odour…and can lead to hyperacidity within the organism.

An adult's daily requirement is 35 ml per kg of body weight – equivalent to 2.5 litres for an adult weighing 65 kg. The requirement increases in high temperatures, with physical activity or with raised body temperature.

It's beneficial to drink about a litre of water (preferably still mineral or spring water) before the middle of the day. Then the body is better able to excrete waste materials. If you drink large amounts of water only in the afternoon or evening, it puts strain on the heart and kidneys.

Water is fundamentally the best mode of transport for cleaning toxins out of the body. In order to meet the body's fluid requirements, you should drink lots of water every day. Fruit and vegetable juices without added sugar, best of all freshly squeezed, are also recommended on a daily basis for their high vitamin content. There is also the choice of herbal teas, preferably unsweetened, but if not, with honey. Ground coffee and black tea are addictive and should be drunk only in moderation. They don't count as part of a person's daily fluid requirements. Coffee and alcoholic drinks draw moisture out of body tissue, therefore they should not count towards daily intake.

Water and other drinks should not be drunk ice cold straight from the fridge, as ice-cold drinks give a shock to the nerves of the stomach. This can lead to restricted function of the stomach.

Another method of detoxifying the body is to simmer a litre of water for approximately 15–20 minutes over a low heat. Simmering changes the composition and taste of the water and generates healing qualities. Then pour the water into a thermos flask and drink it slowly, a mouthful at a time, over the course of several hours. Regularity counts here – for example, one cupful per hour. If you like, you could add some fresh lemon, which helps the digestion. If you add some ginger to the water (it's best to do this while it's boiling), it helps to detoxify the liver and to neutralize stomach acid.

In many people the sense of thirst diminishes with age. The reason is a difference in concentration of salts, compared to what it was at a younger age. Therefore older people often drink much too little, which accelerates the ageing process. Many manifestations of ageing are the result of wrong drinking habits. In this case you can outwit yourself by setting aside the amount of fluid your body needs in the morning, and drinking it over the course of the day. If drinking the right amount of water makes you feel better, you will regain your natural sense of thirst.

Avoid drinking with, or immediately after, meals. Do it beforehand, or at the soonest an hour afterwards, as otherwise the digestive juices are diluted and the digestive process is made more difficult for the body. Then subsequently consumed food cannot be digested properly, or in a timely manner. Also, the stomach is overloaded as it tries to bring diluted stomach acid back to normal physiological levels by producing more of it.

Coffee and black tea

There is no objection to the morning cup of coffee or a cosy teatime. Moderation is the word! Caffeine acts as a stimulant on the central nervous system. It is addictive, causes withdrawal symptoms and leads to mental and physical dependency. It leads to raised heart rate, irregular circulation in the coronary blood vessels, high blood pressure, diabetes, kidney failure and stomach ulcers. Further, it draws fluid away from body tissues. It disturbs blood sugar levels, as it makes the pancreas produce insulin.

Coffee and tea are very acid-forming. The more acid in your blood, the more water the body retains in order to dilute the acidity. This puts strain on the organism and causes weight gain.

Decaffeinated coffee is just as acid-forming for the body. The caffeine-removing process demands the use of a highly concentrated solution that penetrates deep inside the coffee bean, and which has to be digested when you drink the coffee. Coffee that has been decaffeinated using steam or other non-chemical means is preferable to chemically decaffeinated coffee.

If, in spite of knowing this, your desire for coffee remains very strong, then try to restrict your coffee intake gradually. You might try a cup of a good coffee substitute. Much of what we consume in the course of a day is pure habit and may also be changed gradually.

Why garlic is healthy

Not only does garlic add that special something to a dish, but our body also benefits from its health-giving influence. The reason is in its high antioxidant properties. Scientists at the University of Bonn have now examined its healing effect and have come to the conclusion that it is sulphurous substances, the so-called allicin, that are transformed by the enzyme allinase into the strong-smelling allicin, and bring about healing. People who eat garlic every day are not only protecting themselves from certain cancers of the stomach and intestinal tract, but also taking care of their heart and circulatory system, for garlic has an anti-arteriosclerotic effect.

The white bulb also reduces raised levels of lipids in the blood, inhibits blood clotting and lowers blood pressure. Chopped garlic kills bacteria and can therefore be regarded as a natural antibiotic. It makes no difference whether you take fresh garlic or garlic capsules, as the sulphur content of both comes within the same range.

To sum up, I want to impress upon you that you should enjoy everything you eat and drink. For example, if you like to eat sweet things, try to do so in moderation, and enjoy it. Regard that cup of coffee not as a sin, but as a pleasure that you grant yourself. Aim to set yourself free from 'bad habits'; just bear in mind that this doesn't happen overnight, but rather one step at a time. Don't be too strict with yourself.

WHY I WROTE THIS BOOK

It was 1993. I had completed my yoga teacher-training at the Rekai School of Yoga in Berlin scarcely two years previously, and was teaching two Hatha yoga courses. At this time a friend of mine, also a yoga teacher, told me that she was offering chair yoga for elderly people. I listened with interest and gladly accepted her invitation to a yoga session with her senior citizens' group. A new world was opened up for me. I discovered how full of variety the chair programme is.

I made contact with Frau Erika Hammerström, who developed chair yoga, visited her and found out how, after years of instructing young people, she came to be working almost exclusively with older people, and also to have developed a programme for chair yoga – full of variety, intensive, with only the slightest risk of doing oneself an injury through difficult exercises, and suitable for those who discover yoga only in their old age or who are not particularly supple.

I gladly accepted Frau Hammerström's notes for teaching chair yoga and took the earliest opportunity to visit her classes. These had great appeal for me. I was touched by the experience of how important their weekly yoga class was for these older participants. Not just because they were doing something for their health – the fact of being linked in to a community and staying in touch with one another also seemed to do all the participants good.

I built up my knowledge more and more, until I too was able to teach it. Over the years the desire grew in me to pass my knowledge on. I put together my experience of this still fairly unknown form of yoga and decided to publish it in a book. Today I am leading ten courses, eight of which, including six courses of chair yoga, are for older people.

I would like to offer my book not only to people who want to do something for their health and are interested in learning chair yoga. I would also like to offer it to yoga teachers who wish to work with older or disabled people and are looking for a suitable alternative to classical yoga on a mat. For them, perhaps my book will act as a pointer to opening up to something new and to give more older or disabled people the opportunity of doing something regularly for their physical and mental health.

INDEX

abdominal muscles, exercises for people
    with strong 50, 51–2
Adham Pranayama (inferior front part of
    lungs) 22
Adhyam Pranayama (superior front part of
    lungs) 24
Ahimsa (non-violence) 170
animal medication 181
Aparigraha (non-possessiveness) 171–2
ardour 173
Arjuna (warrior) 169–70
arms
    awareness of and benefits of exercises 71
    exercises for 73–89
Asanas 96–7, 174
    see also poses and postures
Asteya (not stealing) 171
Atman Pranidad (devotion to God) 174

back
    awareness of and benefits of exercises
        91–2
    exercises for 93–106
balancing pose exercise 137
being-at-one 15, 175–6
bending exercises 46, 68, 94, 105
Bhagavad Gita 169–70
bicycling exercise 50
black tea 184, 185
boat pose exercise 53–4
Brahma Danda (spine) 91–2
Brahma Mudra (turning the head slowly)
        116–17
brain
    exercises for 133–8
    hemispheres of 131–2

Bramacharya (control of sensuality) 171
breath control
    effects of correct and incorrect 20
    energy 19–20
    exercises for 22–31
    and lungs 21
breath, extension of 174
bud exercise 66

cautionary notes 50, 72, 96, 98, 103, 115,
    128
cereal 179
chair yoga
    how best to begin 16–17
    requirements 14
    structure of exercises 14–15
    suitable for 14
chair yoga programmes
    fifteen-minute 156–8
    forty-five-minute 161–6
    planning 155–6
    sixty-minute 166–7
    text to lead a group 154
    thirty-minute 158–61
chest widening exercise 76
circling exercises 47, 62, 73–4, 111–12,
        118, 126, 127, 128, 148
circulation exercises
    feet 36, 40, 41
    general 49, 50, 53, 123
    hands 61, 64, 66
    legs 45
'clang' exercise 133
clapping exercises 49, 86
clothing 20
coffee 184, 185

composure 175
concentration 175
   exercises for 24, 63, 76, 98, 136, 148
conscious relaxation 152–3
contentment 173
crane exercise 123–4
crescent moon exercise 121–2
crossing arms exercise 78

dance pose exercise 93
Dharana (concentration/composure) 175
diet 176–7, 186
   black tea and coffee 185
   correct diet 177
   effects of bad nutrition 180
   garlic 185–6
   meat eating 180
   nuts 183
   organic foods 178
   seed sprouts 181–2
   sugar 182–3
   water 184–5
   whole foods 179–80
discipline, spiritually motivated 173
Dola Dolati (variation on standing twist)
   129–30
dropping the shoulders exercise 110
Dyana (meditation) 175

ecstasy 175–6
'eight-fold path' 170–6
elbows, extending exercise 75
energy, extension of 174
exercises, general rules for 18
extension exercises 75, 99–100, 105, 106
eyes
   awareness of 143–4
   benefits of exercises 144
   exercises for 145–50

feet
   awareness of 33–4
   benefits of exercises 34
   exercises for 35–42
fibre 180
fingers
   awareness of and benefits of exercises
      55–6

exercises for 57–9, 61–4, 66
fist exercises 64, 66
food *see* diet
full yogic breathing exercise 25

garlic 185–6
generosity 171–2
God, devotion to 174
'gong' exercise 134

half moon exercise 121–2
half spinal twist exercise 96–7
hand-to-knee cross-patterning exercise 136
hands
   awareness of and benefits of exercises
      55–6
   exercises for 57–69
harmonizing exercise 80–2
Hatha yoga 175–6
head exercises 115, 116–17, 146–7
heel exercises 35, 42, 47
higher awareness 175
hips
   artificial 96, 103
   circling exercise 127
horizontal figure of eight exercise 138

inner fire, developing 173
inner vision 173–4

knee exercises 44, 126
Kollath, W.G. 180

lateral extension exercise 105
legs
   awareness of and benefits of exercises 43
   exercises for 44–54
loosening exercises 39, 83
lungs
   inferior front part 22
   lobes of 21
   lower side and back region 26
   middle front part 23
   middle side and back region 27
   superior front part 24
   upper side and back region 28
lymph flow stimulation exercises 51–2, 94,
   105

Madhyam Pranayama (middle front part of lungs) 23
Mahat Mudra (breathing into separate parts of lungs) 22–4, 26–8
Mahat Yoga Pranayama (full yogic breathing) 25
massaging exercises 45, 113, 146
Matsyendra Asana (half spinal twist) 96–7
meat 180
meditation 175
milling 179
mountain pose exercise 84–5

Namaskara Mudra (harmonizing exercise) 80–2
Natarajasana (dance pose) 93
Nava Kriya (boat pose variation) 53–4
Navasana (boat pose variation) 53–4
neck
    awareness of and benefits of exercises 107–8
    exercises for 109–18
Niyamas (observances) 172–4
non-possessiveness 171–2
non-stealing 171
non-violence 170
nostrils, breathing exercise 30–1
nutrition *see* diet
nuts 183

observances 172–4
opening the hands exercise 65
organic foods 178

'PAH' exercise 83
Pavanmuktasana (wind-releasing exercise) 48
pelvic floor
    anatomy 139
    exercises for 139–40, 141
    tips for 140
'pendulum' exercise 129–30
poses and postures 174
    exercises 53–4, 84–5, 93, 137
Prana (divine energy) 19–20
Pranayama (extension of breath/energy) 174
    see also breath control
Pratyahara (withdrawal of the senses) 174

present, being in the 17
pressing exercises 58, 60
propeller exercise 109
proteins 180
purity 172–3
pushing exercises 44, 88, 89

raising exercises 35, 135
relaxation 151–2
    exercise 152–3
restrictions, general 170–2
ribcage relaxing exercise 77
rocking on soles exercise 36
rolling the feet exercise 37
roughage 179

Samadhi (being-at-one/ecstasy) 175–6
Santosha (contentment) 173
Satya (truth) 171
Saucha (purity) 172–3
Savitri Pranayama (breathing exercise) 29–30
seeds 181–2
self-knowledge 173–4
senses, withdrawal of 174
sensuality, control of 171
Shiva 169–70
shoulders
    awareness of and benefits of exercises 107–8
    exercises for 109–18
smokers, advice for 17
soles, rocking exercise 36
spinal twist exercises
    with arms bent 101–2
    half spinal twist 96–7
    with outstretched arms 103–4
    standing twist variation 129–30
    twisting forward bend 94–5
spine 91–2
standing exercises 121–30
    benefits of 120
    correct posture for 119
stress 15, 16, 151
stretching exercises 41, 69, 79, 87, 114
sugar 182–3
Surya Bhedana Pranayama (alternate nostril breathing) 31–2
Swadhyaya (self-knowledge through inner vision) 173–4

Tapas (developing inner fire) 173
tea 184, 185
throat *see* neck
tiger breathing exercise 98
toes, exercises for 38–40, 42
truth 171
twisting exercises *see* spinal twist exercises

upper body, exercises for 44, 84–5, 88, 89,
	109, 128

varicose veins 43
	prevention exercises 35, 36

waking up the feet exercise 38
walking exercises 42, 125
watching a pendulum exercise 149
water 184–5
whole foods 179–80
wind-releasing exercise 48
withdrawal of the senses 174
World Health Organization 182
wrists, exercises for 57, 64, 67–9

Yamas (general restrictions) 170–2
yoga
	benefits of 15–16
	history of 13–14, 169–70